THE
PSYCHEDELIC
FUTURE
OF THE
MIND

"With intelligence, keen insight, deep knowledge, and a wonderful ability to imagine a future illuminated by the powerful interaction between entheogens and the seeking human mind, Thomas Roberts pulls off a visionary book about the most fascinating subject imaginable."

TOM SHRODER, AUTHOR OF *OLD SOULS*
AND *FIRE ON THE HORIZON*

"Tom Roberts is one of the few elder statesmen of the psychedelic world concerned with the inevitable social and medical repercussions arising from the continued worldwide use and growing medical and governmental acceptance of entheogens. I find his speculations and their implications wise and innovative."

JAMES FADIMAN, PH.D., AUTHOR OF
THE PSYCHEDELIC EXPLORERS GUIDE

"Roberts's work in the area of entheogens—man's use of psychedelic substances in the context of religious rite or spiritual growth—has sought to replace popular uninformed hysteria with actual facts and, through critical examination, illuminate the ways in which our brains process and interpret our perceptions. He has earned his place among the best inner explorers of our time."

"Roberts's book is a tour de force in the nascent field of psychedelic studies. *The Psychedelic Future of the Mind* proposes bold new research directions and methodologies that intrepidly advance what psychedelic research can become. A guide for researchers and the general public alike, this book promotes paths to integrate the power of psychedelic insights into both careers and daily life."

THE
PSYCHEDELIC
FUTURE
OF THE
MIND

How Entheogens Are Enhancing
Cognition, Boosting Intelligence,
and Raising Values

THOMAS B. ROBERTS, PH.D.

Park Street Press
Rochester, Vermont • Toronto, Canada

Park Street Press
One Park Street
Rochester, Vermont 05767
www.ParkStPress.com

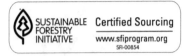

Text stock is SFI certified

Park Street Press is a division of Inner Traditions International

Library of Congress Cataloging-in-Publication Data

Roberts, Thomas B.
  The psychedelic future of the mind : how entheogens are enhancing cognition, boosting intelligence, and raising values / Thomas B. Roberts.
    p. cm.
  Includes bibliographical references and index.
  Summary: "Explores scientific and medical research on the emerging uses of psychedelics to enrich mind, morals, spirituality, and creativity"—Provided by publisher.
  ISBN 978-1-59477-459-1 (pbk.) — ISBN 978-1-59477-502-4 (e-book)
  1. Altered states of consciousness. 2. Hallucinogenic drugs—Psychological aspects. I. Title.
  QP360.R58 2013
  612.8—dc23
                                                                    2012019794

Printed and bound in the United States by Lake Book Manufacturing, Inc. The text stock is SFI certified. The Sustainable Forestry Initiative® program promotes sustainable forest management.

10 9 8 7 6 5 4 3 2 1

Text design by Jack Nichols and layout by Brian Boynton
This book was typeset in Garamond Premier Pro with Futura and Gill Sans used as display typefaces

To send correspondence to the author of this book, mail a first-class letter to the author c/o Inner Traditions • Bear & Company, One Park Street, Rochester, VT 05767, and we will forward the communication.

With love to Susan and Becca.

You are my sunlight and sky, my clover leaf and pine.

This Is My Song
(To be sung to the tune "Finlandia")

This is my song, O God of all the nations,
A song of peace for lands afar and mine:
This is my home, the country where my heart is.
Here are my hopes, my dreams, my holy shrine.

But other hearts in other lands are beating,
With hopes and dreams as true and high as mine.

My country's skies are bluer than the ocean,
And sunlight beams on clover leaf and pine.
But other lands have sunlight, too, and clover,
And skies are everywhere as blue as mine.

O hear my song, O God of all the nations,
A song of peace for their land and for mine.

LLOYD STONE

Contents

A Note to Readers   ix

Introduction: A Short Trail Guide to This Book   1

PART 1

THE EXPERIENCE THAT ALTERS ALL OTHERS

1   Our Psychedelic Future   7

2   Humanity's Taproot   13

3   Raising Values   37

4   The New Religious Era   55

5   Psychedelics and Religious Experiences—What Is the
    Relationship? by Roger N. Walsh, M.D., Ph.D., D.H.L.   80

6   Do Psychedelic-induced Mystical Experiences
    Boost the Immune System?   88

7   Psychedelic Psychotherapy Near the End of Life
    by Charles S. Grob, M.D., and Alicia L. Danforth   102

PART 2

HIGH-YIELD IDEAS—MULTISTATE THEORY
AND THE FRUITFUL MIND

8   Multistate Theory—Apps Are to Devices
    as Mindbody States Are to Minds   121

9   Enhancing Cognition, Boosting Intelligence,
Expanding Cognitive Studies   135

10   New Intellectual Endeavors   146

11   It's a Perinatal World—Hitler and War, Sartre
and Mescaline, *Snow White* and *Fight Club*   159

12   The Neurosingularity Project—When Bigger
Heads and Better Brains Surpass Our Current Ones   178

PART 3

FROM LAB TO LIFE, FROM CLINIC TO CAMPUS

13   Reaching the Unreachable Public While Raising
$1+ Billion for Psychedelic R & D via Crowdfunding—
A Biz-fi Speculation   193

14   It Means Something Different to be Well Educated   207

15   You Teach *What? Where?*   220

Conclusion: Hopes   232

Appendix: Community Psychedelic Centers
International, Inc.—Notes for a Prospectus   235

References   247

Index   267

A Note to Readers

From my own experiences and through readings I have become increasingly respectful of the power of LSD and other psychedelic drugs. Like any powerful thing, they can be destructive or constructive, depending on how skillfully they are used. Among other things, they can concentrate your attention on the most vulnerable, most unpleasant parts of your mind. Therefore, psychedelic drugs should be explored only under the guidance of a qualified guide, one who has extensive psychedelic training. If you need assistance, most mental health professionals may be of little help, and some could even worsen your state, as they are currently mistrained concerning psychedelics.

Furthermore, street dosages are of unknown strength and questionable purity. Until the time you can explore your mind using psychedelics of known strength and purity under qualified guidance, within the law, I urge you to limit yourself to studying the literature and working within professional and other organizations for the resumption of legal, scientific, religious, or academic research.

A Short Trail Guide to This Book

This book looks forward, not backward. Experiences beget ideas, and *The Psychedelic Future of the Mind* is an exploration of some ideas psychedelics engender. Based upon a collection of pieces of scientific research, case studies, anecdotes, and other information about psychedelics, this book asks, "When all these pieces are assembled, what do they tell us about what it means to be a human, about our minds, and about the future?"

Our answers will necessarily be partial, because their implications for what it means to be fully human and for what our society is are long and complicated. As researchers complete new studies, tomorrow's findings will refine today's tentative ones. Some future discoveries will correct our errors. Others will confirm and elaborate our current views. And yet others will give birth to ideas we have not even thought of yet.

This is not a book about the discovery and history of LSD and all the strange and wonderful characters who are part of that story.

This is not a book about psychotherapy and the seemingly miraculous cures psychedelics sometimes produce.

This is not a book about how psychedelics plug in to receptor sites on neurons and set the brain adancing.

This is not a book of the I-drank-ayahuasca-puked-and-saw-the-anaconda-goddess kind.

In a real sense, this book follows Jacob Bronowski's (1976) recipe in *The Ascent of Man* for how to speculate in order to advance knowledge: "That's the essence of science: Ask the impertinent question, and you are on your way to pertinent science." The questions embedded in this book are leads that deserve to be followed in more depth. The personal anecdotes and experimental findings reported here both stimulate these questions and are beginnings of answers, but we need additional evidence to answer the questions more conclusively, or even a bit more firmly.

I find it handy to think of the benefits of psychedelics as falling into two broad groups: mediating mystical experiences and revealing previously unknown aspects of our minds. Mystical experiences are powerful and overwhelming. They temporarily give a sense of setting aside one's identification with oneself, often with the realization of being a strand woven in a complex tapestry of perception, insight, and emotions. However, psychedelics can provide a different kind of experience, in which they give us access to the unconscious parts of our minds. They amplify events in our minds that are usually below our awareness so that we can become aware of them. I think the word *psychomagnifiers* fits them well.

These two categories parallel the two aspects of psychedelic psychotherapy identified by Stanislav Grof (1975, 1980): 1) powerful, emotionally positive, peak-experience *psychedelic* psychotherapy; and 2) less-powerful emotion-exploring *psycholytic* psychotherapy. The first uses large doses of psychedelics with the intent of producing a mystical experience. The latter uses lower doses to help people bring emotionally charged hidden events into consciousness.

Unlike many quieter mindbody* states, mystical experiences shout so loudly we cannot ignore them. Part 1 of *The Psychedelic Future of the Mind* examines mystical experiences, with an emphasis on psychedelic effects, and listens to their message.

---

*In this context the one combined word *mindbody* is preferable, because it conveys the concept of mind and body as one, combined, unified whole.

Part 2 is a rough parallel to psycholytic psychotherapy, but it pays more attention to the cognitive aspects of lower-dose sessions rather than to their intensely emotional effects, seeing psychedelics as tools to think with rather than focusing on their psychotherapeutic potential. Emotions and thinking constantly affect each other, of course. They are not divided by a wall but are twins from the same womb of our unconscious, albeit not identical twins.

In part 3 we will explore how the experience that alters all others can lead to a new business and also consider how it expands what it means to be well educated.

PART 1: THE EXPERIENCE THAT ALTERS ALL OTHERS

Part 1 begins our idea-journey into psychedelic mystical experiences. We will stop along the way to:

- compare psychedelic mystical experiences with nonpsychedelic ones
- look at how these experiences affect values
- recognize a new religious era based on direct personal experiences rather than words
- speculate that they may boost our immune systems
- be relieved to know that they can reduce our fear of death

PART 2: HIGH-YIELD IDEAS

Mystical experiences are only one instance of many overall shifts in the ways we perceive, think, feel, and act—many other mindbody states. In part 2 our path takes us to a bluff overlooking a wider prospect, and we see other paths into the psychogeography of our minds. This wider vision embeds psychedelics in a more general Multistate Theory, which helps organize how we think about our mind while it guides us to new ideas. Relying again on psychedelic examples, the path through part 2 shows us psychedelics can—but do not always:

- enhance cognition and raise intelligence
- guide us toward new intellectual frontiers
- produce new ways to interpret history, philosophy, and movies
- even suggest that we can design new thinking processes

Stretching the visionary sense even more, the last chapter of part 2 speculates about improving the brains of future generations.

PART 3: FROM LAB TO LIFE, FROM CLINIC TO CAMPUS

In part 3 our psychedelic idea-hike leads us into a town of the future. How can society benefit from the ideas we have discovered along the psychedelic trail? We will glance at planning-stage, hopeful ideas for:

- raising $1 billion or more for psychedelic research and development
- recruiting the public to support uses of psychedelics
- founding a new business to provide safe, professionally guided psychedelic sessions
- reframing "well educated" to include learning to access useful abilities that reside in various mindbody states
- enriching academia with new research questions, specialties, methods, and courses and course content

I hope every chapter will sprout fresh ideas in your mind.

PART I

The Experience That Alters All Others

Could there really be an experience that alters our lives, not in a traumatic sense, but in positive ways? In *Psychedelic Drugs Reconsidered,* Lester Grinspoon, M.D., and James Bakalar, J.D., then both on the staff of the Harvard Medical School's Department of Psychiatry, put it this way, "It is assumed that if, as is often said, one traumatic event can shape a life, one therapeutic event can reshape it" (1979, 195). While their judgment was about psychotherapy, this part of *The Psychedelic Future of the Mind* extends their comment to other features of our daily lives. The values we live by, spiritual growth, our immune systems, and death are major factors in our lives, and here we explore how mystical experiences can change them.

The first chapter begins with a review of recent publications, which make it clear that research regarding the benefits of psychedelics is, as one of the titles puts it, "making a comeback." From the point of view of the human mind and society, psychedelics' most amazing effects occur when they produce mystical experiences—mystical in the sense of religious experience, not mystical in the sense of "spooky" or "Halloweeny." As a basis for our further explorations, we will describe mystical experiences—both nonpsychedelic and psychedelic—in chapter 2. These descriptions provide background information for the subsequent chapters in part 1, where we examine what current experimental, clinical-laboratory psychedelic research says about our minds, lives, and society.

As chapter 3 illustrates, psychedelic-induced mystical experiences offer a grand feast for ethicists. Mystical experiences often—but by no means always—help people shift away from I-me-mine values of self-centeredness toward values that emphasize social responsibility and spiritual motivation. From mystical roots of changed values we will move on to examine the mystical roots of "the new religious era" in chapter 4.

Psychiatrist Roger Walsh, guest author of chapter 5, addresses the challenge of how to make the insights gained from psychedelic mystical experiences part of our lives. Chapter 6 speculates that mystical experiences might substantially boost our immune systems and proposes that researchers investigate this idea. Part 1 ends with another guest chapter, by psychiatrist Charles Grob and his coresearcher Alicia Danforth, in which they present their research that underlines what I expect will be one of the first widely accepted uses of psychedelics: reducing the fear of death in people with terminal illness whose death is immanent.

1

Our Psychedelic Future

Virtually all current psychedelic research is done in a medical-psychotherapeutic context, as is demonstrated by the chapters Michael Winkelman and I collected from most of the world's leading psychedelic medical researchers, published as our two-book set, *Psychedelic Medicine: New Evidence for Hallucinogenic Substances as Treatments* (2007). The applications of psychedelics identified by our authors were primarily medical and life enhancing. The curative applications included post-traumatic stress disorder, cluster headaches, obsessive-compulsive disorder, facing inner fears, marriage and relationship problems, depression, HIV-AIDS, existential anxiety, fear of death, neuroses and psychoses, alcoholism, and addictions.

Hidden among the health-enhancing applications, we can spot nuggets of spiritual significance, personal meaning, psychological growth, and self-understanding. Sometimes these benefits were not explicitly stated, but lurked in the background. Their observations point out our need to fill in the gaps in our awareness of the uses and implications of psychedelics. A good start has already been made in religion-spirituality, but the work so far mostly lags behind that in medicine. The publications in the arts and humanities are rich in provocative ideas but lack a systematic approach.

WHY NOW?

Psychedelics have been lurking underground in science since the mid-1960s. Is this the time to bring them back above ground for more careful scientific scrutiny? Judging from professional publications, apparently so. In addition to a swarm of Internet sites devoted to psychedelics, a flock of articles in professional scientific journals and general magazines recommend reconsidering them. Among them, six esteemed publications express the tone of the current rediscovery of psychedelics.

- *The Chronicle of Higher Education*. "Researchers Explore New Visions for Hallucinogens." "After a long hiatus, medical investigators return to studying the benefits of once-banned compounds" (Brown 2006).
- *The Lancet*. "Research on Psychedelics Moves into the Mainstream" (Morris 2008, 1491–92).
- *American Psychological Association Monitor*. "Research on Psychedelics Makes a Comeback" (Novotney 2010, 10).
- *Scientific American*. "Hallucinogens as Medicine" (Griffiths and Grob 2010, 76–79).
- *The Economist*. "Acid Tests. Research into Hallucinogenic Drugs Begins to Shake Off Decades of Taboo" (2010, June 23).
- *The New York Times Magazine*. "Is the World Ready for Medical Hallucinogens?—A Kaleidoscope at the End of the Tunnel" (Slater 2012, 56–60, 66).

The Chronicle of Higher Education is a widely circulated weekly newspaper subscribed to by professors, administrators, and others in colleges, universities, and research institutes. It is the newspaper of record for higher education. Its 2006 article was largely in response to a study at Johns Hopkins Medical Institute on psilocybin-induced mystical-type experiences in laboratory conditions. In a very real sense, the Hopkins study broke the ice for news media to publish other psychedelic findings. It was reported on in more than three hundred newspapers, national TV news broadcasts, websites, and magazines, and continues to be cited often in professional journals. The original study with commentaries and two follow-up studies, along with a list and links to news reports, are at the website of the Council on Spiritual Practices: www .csp.org/psilocybin.

The Lancet is certainly one of the world's most prestigious journals of general medicine. If something appears in *The Lancet,* it is probably worthy of note, and the article's title, "Research on Psychedelics Moves into the Mainstream," reflects the shift in attitudes toward psychedelics during the twenty-first century. The author, Kelly Morris, had previously published an editorial, "Hallucinogen Research Inspired Neurotheology" (2006), in *The Lancet*'s sister publication, *The Lancet Neurology*. Her article in May 2008 reported on a World Psychedelic Forum held in March of that year in Basel, Switzerland. More than two thousand people from over forty nations attended it and a similar conference held in 2006. The meetings, she reports, showed a "more measured attitude of researchers toward the risks and benefits of drugs like lysergide (LSD), psilocybin, and methylenedioxymethamfetamine (MDMA)."

Professional groups are catching this rising tide too. At the August 2010 annual meeting of the American Psychological Association, MAPS (the Multidisciplinary Association for Psychedelic Studies) organized a panel discussion on the treatment of post-traumatic stress disorder and on death anxiety. The expansion of psychedelics beyond medicine also received support. "While Dr. Schuster was happy to see psychedelic research being conducted for specific psychiatric purposes," wrote MAPS deputy director Valerie Mojeiko, "he also actively advocated for exploration into the potential application of psychedelics for spiritual and personal growth and development—quite a refreshing perspective from a former [National Institute of Drug Abuse] Director!" (2010, 18).

Following up on the meeting, in November 2010 the American Psychological Association's monthly publication for its 150,000 members, *The Monitor,* noted psychedelics as making a "comeback." Appropriately, the author, Amy Novotney (2010, 10), points out that the FDA and the Drug Enforcement Administration have eased regulations. At the same time, unlike some research decades ago, in all current studies there are firm medical and psychiatric standards for volunteer subjects to meet, careful screening, exact doses and procedures, and thorough preparation and follow-up. The standards include standby medical and psychological assistance if needed. Current research has to obtain approval of institutional review boards as well as the federal agencies. Psychedelics are not prescribed and taken home, but are administered in comfortable clinical settings with professional monitors attending during the full-day sessions.

For general readers who like to keep informed of advances in science, *Scientific American* is one of the forefront publications. It is the oldest continuously published magazine in the United States, has fourteen foreign-language editions, and is distributed in thirty countries as well as online. Its articles are professionally vetted, so when its more than five million readers found "Hallucinogens as Medicine" in the December 2010 issue, psychedelic research had made it to the scientifically informed public. The research projects of the two authors—Roland Griffiths (2006, 2008, 2011) at Johns Hopkins and Charles Grob (2007, 2011) of UCLA Medical Center—though primarily oriented toward psychotherapy, have significant implications for how we understand our minds, and they offer opportunities for improving society.

The internationally renowned magazine *The Economist* covers much more than money, business, and securities. Available worldwide, its expert writers are among the top in their fields, and when it reports that decades of taboo are being shaken off, that opens the eyes and minds of informed general readers.

When the *New York Times,* one of the world's premier newspapers, carried an article about psychedelic medicine in its April 22, 2012, magazine section, many people in the psychedelic field felt that it was an announcement to the general public of the respectability of their professional expertise.

A clear message of the professional acceptability of psychedelic explorations had previously come in April 2010 at *Psychedelic Science in the Twenty-first Century,* a conference organized by the Multidisciplinary

Association for Psychedelic Studies in collaboration with the Heffter Research Institute, the Council on Spiritual Practices, and the England-based Beckley Foundation. Doctors, medical professionals, social workers, and psychologists could obtain continuing education credits for their respective professions by attending a specific track of meetings during this conference; they can still do so by watching the videos online (www.spiritualcompetency.com). The conference was so popular that organizers had to stop accepting registrations and turned people away. An extensive video library is available at www.maps.org/media/videos.

As figure 1.1 demonstrates, several arts, sciences, and humanities are involved in the study of psychedelics.

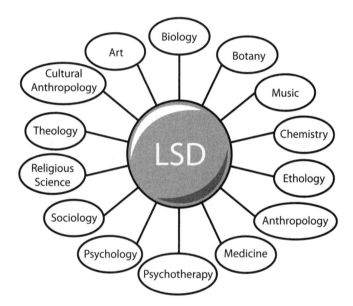

Figure 1.1. Sciences involved in the study of LSD and other hallucinogens. From: Hintzen and Passie (2010) The Pharmacology of LSD. Courtesy of the Beckley Foundation.

WHERE DO WE GO FROM HERE?

Current academic advances indicate that higher education is awakening to psychedelics' opportunities for the world of ideas. Until recently the booming field of positive psychology had ignored psychedelic research, but the second edition of *Positive Psychology: The Science of Happiness and Flourishing* (Compton and Hoffman 2012) includes: 1) peak experiences, 2) meditation and Eastern psychology, 3) transpersonal psychology, 4) mysticism, 5) contemplative spirituality, and 6) entheogens. Congratulations to the authors and publisher. Chapter 15 describes current psychedelic courses at a community college, a university, a medical school, and elsewhere, so things are looking up.

The University of Pennsylvania exercised leadership in the broader academic world in September 2012 with an interdisciplinary conference Psychedemia. "Psychedemia" is an amalgam of "psychedelic" and "academia." In addition to sessions on psychotherapy that are common at psychedelic research meetings, attendees from China and Australia to Brazil and the Czech Republic considered art, ethics, the humanities, personality change, well-being, religion, shamanism, and library archives as well as a film screening and an art exhibit.

As the articles mentioned above make clear, the use of psychedelics in medicine, especially psychotherapy, is getting the most research and media attention. After decades of hibernation, psychedelic psychotherapy is now striding toward treating a variety of human problems. But study of the cultural benefits of psychedelics lags behind. A good start has already been made in studies related to applications in religion and spirituality, but several other nonpsychotherapeutic applications deserve greater attention. I hope *The Psychedelic Future of the Mind* will help awaken more active cultural curiosity.

2

Humanity's Taproot

Do you remember—or can you imagine—how you and your world changed when you went through puberty? You became interested in new things. You saw meanings that you had not seen before in movies, TV shows, humor, advertising, and things you read. Sex became an interest and a motivation. Relationships rose in importance. Puberty altered almost everything else. In many ways you became a new person. Puberty isn't the only such wide-ranging, life-changing event. Mystical experiences cause a similar wide-ranging shift.

Near the beginning of the "psychedelic sixties," Wilson Van Dusen, chief clinical psychologist at Mendocino State Hospital in Talmage, California, described the impact of mystical experiences in his article "LSD and the Enlightenment of Zen."

> There is a central human experience which alters all other experiences . . . so central that men have spent their lives in search of it. Once found, life is altered because the very root of human identity has been deepened. I wish to draw attention to the fact that the still experimental drug d-lysergic acid diethylamide (LSD) appears to facilitate the discovery of this apparently ancient and universal experience. (1961, 11)

What is this experience? How does it change people? Can LSD actually make it more likely to occur? Are mystical experiences that come via drugs really legitimate; do they have the same effect, or are they pale facsimiles, mere imitations of, genuine ones?

MYSTICAL EXPERIENCES

Unfortunately the word *mystical* as we use it in our ordinary language has a vague meaning quite different from its use in religion and psychology. To most people the word *mystical* suggests weird happenings, ghosts, odd "forces" or "beings," strangeness, inexplicable events, scariness, and a sense of dread. An imaginary movie title such as *Three-headed Zombies from Outer Space Invade Area 51* might be described as *mystical* in a trailer or TV listing. This common meaning is quite different from the use of the word in religious studies. Wainwright clarifies this difference succinctly in *Mysticism: A Study of Its Nature, Cognitive Value, and Moral Implications*.

> Mystical experiences should be distinguished from ordinary religious feelings and sentiments, from numinous experiences, and from visions, voices and such occult phenomena as telepathy, clairvoyance, and precognition. None of these experiences is unitary. (1981, 1)

In religion as well as in scholarly circles, an experience is mystical if it shows a particular cluster of subjective experiences. Often the cluster is described as having nine ingredients: unity, transcendence of time and space, deeply felt positive mood, sense of sacredness, objectivity and reality, perspective (or paradoxicality), alleged ineffability, transiency, and persisting changes in attitude or behavior. As is usual in the social sciences and humanities, however, there is always some discussion about how many characteristics a perfect example of something must have, exactly what they are, and whether additional ones should be included.

How many ingredients must be present for an experience to qualify as mystical, and how strong do they need to be? I find it handy to think of a mystical experience as analogous to minestrone: no set recipe but with various combinations of ingredients, and it's the overall taste that matters. While the discussion below describes each characteristic separately, during a mystical experience they are never experienced one at a time. As in soup, each ingredient interacts with all the others. The experience of, say, transcendence flavors the experiences of all the other ingredients, such as mood, unity, sacredness, and so forth.

I had a hard time remembering the nine basic qualities, so I challenged my Psychedelic Studies class to come up with a good mnemonic device for remembering them. In some mnemonic devices such as the planets of the solar system and colors of the rainbow, order is important, but it isn't for mystical experiences. After they worked in small groups for a while, one woman came up with POTT MUSIC: paradoxicality, objectivity, transcendence, transience, mood (deeply felt and positive), unity, sacredness, ineffability, changes.

POTT MUSIC—THE NINE INGREDIENTS OF MYSTICAL EXPERIENCES

In order to gain a deeper understanding of each of these nine characteristics, as well as a closer look at the similarities between naturally occurring mystical experiences and those mediated by psychedelics, we will compare statements recorded in two publications. The naturally occurring instances were published in *Quantum Change* (Miller and C'de Baca 2001). The book, which is subtitled *When Epiphanies and Sudden Insight Transform Ordinary Lives,* came about when William R. Miller, a clinical psychologist and distinguished professor of psychology and psychiatry at the University of New Mexico, noticed a sudden shift for the better in his teenage daughter. Then a friend of his told Miller of a sudden, powerful, and vivid event that changed his life.

These experiences reminded Miller of changes such as Ebenezer Scrooge's in Dickens's *A Christmas Tale* and George Bailey's in the movie *It's a Wonderful Life.* "Their stories seem to rekindle hope in us, even hope against hope—the vision that new life is possible even and especially when it seems most impossible. Entrenched greed turns to generosity. Exuberant joy ignites from the ashes of ruin" (Miller and C'de Baca 2001, 4). He began to wonder: What are these changes? How do they happen? Are they rare or common? What effects did they produce? Miller found little about such experiences in standard psychological literature, so he decided to try to answer these questions himself.

When Miller began, it was in the same spirit that opens each new field of scientific research, the first step often being when someone notices something curious. While scientists usually have some degree of curiosity, curiosity strong enough to notice something new is less common. Most scientific curiosity fits with an existing paradigm—a standard way of thinking about things. The current dominant paradigm typically determines what research most often gets funded, published, and produces promotions. It is "thinking inside the box."

For groundbreaking scientists such as Miller, the second step in scientific research—description—consists of: 1) collecting samples of the curious event or object; 2) finding out how often it happens (frequency count); 3) describing it, eventually resulting in listing the characteristics that an ideal specimen must have; and 4) determining if different types of the thing exist (a typology). In Miller's case he interested a reporter for the *Albuquerque Journal* in writing a story, then he and his coauthor, Janet C'de Baca, interviewed fifty-five respondents who had experienced what Miller and C'de Baca called "quantum changes." They called them this because their interviewees' lives shifted abruptly; they started whole new ways of looking at things. They determined that quantum changes came in two types, insights and epiphanies. For each of the nine POTT MUSIC characteristics, sample statements from *Quantum Change* will provide our nonpsychedelic examples.

They are compared with quotations selected from a paper, "Mystical-type Experiences Occasioned by Psilocybin Mediate the Attribution of Personal Meaning and Spiritual Significance 14 Months Later" (Griffiths et al. 2008), which was a follow-up of an experiment with psilocybin that had been conducted at Johns Hopkins Medical Institute two years previously.* The examples are all from table 3, "Verbatim written comments about the nature of the spiritual experience" (629). In an excellent nineteen-minute *TED* online video, the principal investigator summarizes these reports.

> What I want to tell you about today is some research that demonstrates that psilocybin can occasion, with a very high probability, mystical type experiences that appear virtually identical with naturally occurring mystical experiences as reported by mystics throughout the ages and across different cultures. (Griffiths 2009)

The quotations from *Quantum Change* (Miller and C'de Baca 2001) reflecting transformative epiphanies and sudden insights are labeled "Naturally Occurring" and those from the follow-up of the psilocybin study are labeled "Psychedelically Mediated." They are remarkably similar, both illustrating Van Dusen's observation about "the experience that alters all others."

Paradoxicality of Perspective

Insight, wider understanding, and seeing a broader context often occur during mystical experiences. The new perspective links ideas in new ways, which can solve previously intractable problems. To explain this it is handy to think of mystical experiences as novel information-processing programs that allow the mind to invent new solutions, to see things from a fresh perspective.

During mystical experiences conflicts between opposite ideas appear reduced. They are reframed as complementary aspects of a larger whole, each as part of a more complete view. Similarly, in personal relationships conflicts may be overcome, as the behavior of others becomes more deeply understood. Forgiveness often increases. On a personal level, the broader context of mystical experiences may transform how a person feels about self and others. When Miller and C'de Baca asked

---

*The full article, a table of the volunteers' comments, two associated articles, and more are located at www.csp.org/psilocybin.

their fifty-five interviewees "What was different after your experience?" a common response was, "Everything." "The transformations described were usually at the level of personality, of core guiding principles, of the person's way of perceiving and understanding self and reality" (127).

Naturally Occurring: It's how I look at things and how things are pointed out to me that has changed. (127)

Psychedelically Mediated: The feeling of joy and sadness at the same time—paradoxical. (629)

In his *Varieties of Religious Experience,* the founder of the scientific study of mysticism, early-twentieth-century American philosopher-psychologist William James, expressed this as the "keynote" of mystical experiences—he called it "reconciliation." "It is as if the opposites of the world, whose contradictoriness and conflict make all our difficulties and troubles, were melted into unity" (1958, 298). This contributes to what he calls "metaphysical significance."

Objectivity

The sense that one is in touch with a reality that is realer than in ordinary experience is common. James described this as a state "of insight into depths of truth unplumbed by the discursive intellect" (293). He called this a "noetic quality." *Noetic* comes from the same Greek root as *knowledge,* referring to ideas that are felt as absolutely true, "truer than true," profound, earthshaking, even enlightening. Some noetic experiences have to do with truth, reality, and the nature of the world. Others are more personal, insights aimed at improving one's individual life.

Naturally Occurring: Usually a mystical quantum change includes the experience of being given a message, of having an important truth revealed. This message comes into consciousness with great force and with an immediate sense of certitude. (Miller and C'de Baca 2001, 76)

Psychedelically Mediated: I felt as if tons of information about "what is" was being downloaded quickly into my knowing/understanding. (629)

Just because insights feel cosmically profound does not necessarily mean they are, however. The classic example is questionably attributed to William James. During a nitrous oxide session, he had what seemed to be a key idea to understanding the universe, so he wrote it down (de Ropp 1968, 62). When he returned to his normal state, he found that his cosmically profound statement had turned comically profound.

> *Hogamous, Higamous,*
> *Man is polygamous.*
> *Higamous, Hogamous*
> *Woman is monogamous.*

While not exactly a philosophical breakthrough, James's is not an entirely worthless thought. This is not to say that all noetic truths during mystical experiences are silly, but it cautions us to question mystical insights just as we should our ordinary-state insights.

This raises a curious question about apparently truthful knowledge in both mystical states and our default ordinary state. If the feeling of truth—especially deep, abiding enlightenment—can be "rheostated" up and down as we move from one mindbody state to another, on what grounds can we be most certain about our ideas? Might the sense of truthfulness be just an artifact of our mindbody state—a brain thing, a chemical imbalance? A fascinating opportunity for experimental philosophy opens up: the degree of truthfulness that we feel can change when mindbody states are changed.

Thanks to psychedelics, philosophers can do experiments in which the perception of truthfulness can be a dependent variable. Obviously, our default state is privileged for scientific knowledge, but what state(s) is/are privileged for religious and humanistic knowledge? To enrich their understanding of existing principles and intellectual theories, scholars can test them in various mindbody states—if they dare. Experimental religious studies and experimental humanities are gestating too.

Transcendence

At first leaving our personal identity behind sounds frightening for most people. We like to have a firm sense of who we are, of being in charge of our lives, our thoughts, and our emotions. In fact, getting stuck permanently in an egoless state usually qualifies a person to be considered insane. It comes as a surprise, then, to learn that when one takes off an ego, just as one might take off a jacket or shirt, something remains. People who visit this state and put their self-jacket back on afterward often find it the single most meaningful experience of their lives. How strange it is that leaving one's personhood is personally meaningful! This beyond-the-person experience is the basis for transpersonal psychology (*trans* = "beyond," *personal* = "default identity").

The setting (location or context) and the person's set (psychological state) are major influences on mystical states as a whole and specifically on ego transcendence. The naturally occurring example given below occurred during an experience of great physical pain and resembles others that happened during several accidents. The situation given in the Johns Hopkins follow-up paper was just the opposite. In that study volunteers had been carefully screened, prepared for what to expect, and situated in a comfortable living room–like setting with two supportive monitors.

> *Naturally Occurring:* And then I just felt so at peace. It was very, very, very calming, because I knew something important. I knew I was no longer limited by the physical. I think the pain was so extreme that it forced my consciousness out of my body. I was able to transcend the physical, to see beyond the physical limitations. I have never feared death since then, nor have I ever experienced depression, which was a major change for me. (Miller and C'de Baca 2001, 85)

Psychedelically Mediated: Freedom from every conceivable thing including time, space, relationships, self, etc. . . . . It was as if the embodied "me" experienced ultimate transcendence. (629)

The transcendence of individual identity may shift motivation from the I-me-mine orientation of our normal self-dominant state to a state of wider social responsibility and cosmic awareness. Because one of the fears of death, often unconscious, is giving up the ego, practice sessions of ego transcendence may reduce this anxiety.

Transience

People generally recognize that their mystical experiences are short-lived, take place at a specific time and place, and are different from their ordinary experience. In spite of that, during such an experience time may seem to stand still, or the experience may happen "out of time." It may feel like eternity, or timeless. Entry to a mystical state is often marked by colors appearing brighter and more saturated, music sounding more intense than ever before, and smell and touch being greatly amplified; their decrease to normal intensity marks a return to an ordinary state. Experiencers make references such as "when I came back" or "when it was over," which also indicate a shift from their mystical state to a more ordinary one.

Naturally Occurring: On December 25, 1981, I was driving home from work—Christmas Day. It was approximately 7:30 or 8:00 in the morning. . . . I was driving east on I-40, and all of a sudden I knew it. It just happened. (Miller and C'de Baca 2001, 87)

A different interviewee reported, "Whew! All of a sudden, for about two or three seconds, I had this thing happened to me that was just out of this world." (88)

Psychedelically Mediated: Because the experimental sessions at Johns Hopkins occurred at a set place, at known times and duration, and on certain dates, transience was built into the experiment, so there were no reports of the volunteers mentioning obvious time and place in their subjective accounts. (629)

However, many subjective reports of psychedelic mystical experiences report "coming down" or "returning" that suggest transience (Hayes 2000). Some people experience an afterglow that may last for hours or days. It may or may not influence how they act and experience life afterward. The questions of why people's lives are affected to different degrees and for different lengths of time remain to be answered.

Mood (Deeply Felt, Positive)

After getting over the fears of ego loss, and the general strangeness of mystical experiences, intense positive feelings frequently occur. Ecstasy, love, joy, a profound sense of peace, release from long-term negative emotions, and a sense of gratitude and blessedness are common emotions, frequently at an intensity that the person has never felt before and never believed was possible.

> *Naturally Occurring:* I felt incredible acceptance, love, a sense of well-being, euphoria, everything going to be well. I choose to believe, and I chose to believe at that time, that the presence that was in the car was Jesus Christ. I didn't see him. This was not a visual experience. What I felt was incredible warmth, an incredible sense of well-being. I felt loved like I had never been loved in my life. (Miller and C'de Baca 2001, 87)

> *Psychedelically Mediated:* The utter joy and freedom of letting go—without anxiety—beyond ego self. (629)

The intense positive mood is not a quick flash in the pan. It can transform a person's emotions not just during the experience itself but also enrich the person's life thereafter, providing a more mature and positive outlook.

Naturally Occurring: How has all this changed me? Well, whatever happens, I'm just at peace. I'm not afraid anymore, and I don't think of myself as ugly and dirty and trashy. I'm not afraid of my father. I'm secure and self-assured. I have the patience of a saint now. (128)

Psychedelically Mediated: That in every horrible experience or frightening experience, if you stay with it, enter into it, you will find God. That the horror is in reality only an illusion and God lies beneath it all. It has become a guiding principal in my life. (629)

Which occurs first? Does the intense positive mood make the world feel less threatening, allowing a person to drop fear-based defensiveness to feel connected and united with life? Or, does the sense of unity in the presence of a powerful and loving being outside oneself, "like a baby in a mother's arms," produce the positive emotions? Whichever it is, the combination of positive mood and unity strengthen each other.

Unity

When a psychedelic helps a person to "take off" the sense of self and set it aside, and when a sense of powerful love and peace flows into that person's mind, fear and defensiveness evaporate. The walls between self and other disappear, and people feel at one with an object, a piece of music, a beautiful scene, another person, even with all of humanity or the whole cosmos. Such statements as "I am that" or "I am all things" are not confusion about where one's body ends, but reports of the interconnectedness experienced when the I-me-mine sense of self dissolves.

Naturally Occurring: I felt at peace. I felt reassured. I felt loved too, like there was a union: I was part of something that was a loving peaceful thing, something much larger than me—something loving, something caring, something that was going to take care of [my daughter] too. (83)

Psychedelically Mediated: The feeling of no boundaries—where I didn't know where I ended and my surroundings began. Somehow I was able to comprehend what oneness is. (629)

When people have unitive experiences they gain insight into ideas of the world's religions that include statements such as "We are all one." Unity statements don't mean that we are a mass of separate individuals collected together and acting as a group in concert, but the separation into individuals is itself an illusion. The oneness is analogous to supposing that a cell in the human body were to realize that it is part of the larger body, not just an individual, separated cell. The context of existence is widened. Yet this doesn't prohibit experiencers of unity from functioning as individuals.

When people who have had a mystical experience identify with people who are suffering, say victims of injustice, illness, or privation, they often dedicate themselves to helping others. In doing so, of course, they are relieving the felt pain in themselves too. When ego transcendence is present, the good Samaritan doesn't do his or her loving act for personal gain, nor in order to congratulate himself or herself at being such a fine humane-minded person. Lessening human suffering is simply the way to live one's life.

Sacredness

This is probably the hardest characteristic to understand, not because it is especially rare, but because it's difficult to figure out how to interpret it: the feeling-idea may be free-floating, not attached to anything. Or it may be attached to one specific object. Equally, it might be characteristic of everything: "The whole world is sacred." It is a sense of awe, feeling cared for, being attached to something greater than oneself, even being absorbed in it. Humility and surprised gratitude present the questions, "Why me? Why am I so blessed? What did I do to deserve this great gift?" The experience may or may not be expressed in terms of the experiencer's religion, but there is typically a sense of a Great Loving Other who pours love into the experiencer, deserved or not.

Naturally Occurring: I felt nonjudgmental love. I felt total acceptance for whoever I was. In a spiritual sense, I knew I was not alone, that there was a purpose for the universe, that I was going to be okay. (Miller and C'de Baca 2001, 88)

Psychedelically Mediated: It opened my third eye—I could see many spiritual beliefs that I hold/held and linked them—a more cohesive and comprehensive spiritual landscape became apparent to me. (629)

Ralph Hood (1975, 1993), using his *Mysticism Scale,* the standard instrument for assessing mystical experiences, reported that the sense of sacredness is often missing, so that people can have either a secular mystical experience or a sacred one. This raises wonderfully complex questions: Is sacredness a quality of the experience itself, or is it an interpretation of the experience that the person uses to understand it? In other words, to what extent do our culture, language, ideas, religious background, and society contribute to these experiences, and how much is "raw" experience? When it comes to trying to make sense of mystical experiences, sacredness is the hard seed at the center of this tough nut to crack. Four different approaches can aid our attempt at interpretation: looking at it from the materialist point of view, using analogies, seeing it as projection, and viewing it from the perspective of "creation religion."

Materialism

People with a material view of reality use drug-induced mystical experiences to support their case that religion is merely a delusionary biochemical event in the brain. "If powerful experiences that are called 'religious' can be caused by psychoactive plants and chemicals," they claim, "this just proves that religion is nothing more than a fit of brain craziness that naive believers attach all sorts of odd beliefs to." From this perspective mystical and other religious experiences can be explained away just as dreams are; they are seen as not real in any sense except as subjective experiences. The fact that these plants and chemicals also produce other hallucinations supports their position.

Of course, just because weak electrical currents and drugs can cause a sensation does not mean that there is no reality that can also stimulate similar sensations. Electrical implants in our brains can stimulate sensations of hunger, horniness, or feeling hurt. People would not say that there are no such things as hunger, horniness, or feeling hurt just because they can also be electrically stimulated.

Tuning In to Sacredness and God

A second try at interpreting mystical experiences focuses on how people think about the sacredness ingredient. The analogy of infrared and ultraviolet light plays a useful role here. We know these higher and lower frequencies of light exist but that our optical systems are not tuned to see them. Perhaps the reason we don't see the sacredness of reality is due to the fact that we are not usually tuned to see it. From this perspective, entheogenic* plants and chemicals tune us to see the sacredness that is already there but that we miss. From this perspective, seeing sacredness is a realization: "I was blind, but now I see." Simply, we become aware of what was always there.

An Inside the Brain Event

A third possibility is that we are merely projecting an inner sense of sacredness onto the outside world. Just as a slide projector or movie projector takes a film or digital image and throws it against a screen, our minds make psychological projections by taking an inner feeling or thought and wrongly supposing it comes from the "real" world outside us. For example, when someone is sad, the whole world feels depressive. When we are with the one we love, we project good feelings onto him or her. Probably every adolescent has been disappointed to learn at one time or another that one's projected affection is not returned. Is sacredness an inner feeling that we project onto the world? Most of what we perceive, such as the words on this page or sounds around us, do come to us from the "outside world." It's natural to mistakenly suppose

---

*An *entheogen* is "a chemical substance that is ingested to produce a sacredlike state of consciousness."

that our perception of sacredness is like other sensations, coming from outside us. Do entheogens produce intense inner perceptions that we wrongly suppose come to us through our senses? Or do they alert us to a reality that we would otherwise miss, to a sacredness that surrounds us all the time and everywhere but that we are blind to?

A God-designed Brain

A fascinating yet odd dilemma pertaining to the question of sacredness comes from the perspective of so-called creation religion. According to some creationists, our brains are too complex to have evolved over time, so they must have been created by God. Keeping this assumption in mind and recognizing that human brains have a capacity for mystical experiences, why did God construct our brains so that they can have this experience? If he designed and built our brains with this capacity and we refuse to use it, aren't we practically thumbing our noses at the Almighty? "Sorry, God, we know what to do with our brains better than you do." Why did the creator of all plants design some that would activate our brains into having mystical experiences? I sure don't know.

Ineffability

I enjoy thinking about this trait of mystical experiences because it's so ironic. It is difficult to talk about an experience that is so unlike our ordinary experience, so different that words fail. Yet, after saying that using words is impossible, many experiencers go on to write thousands of words about their experiences. Of course, these descriptions are often analogies—"It was like this, but different"—and they often use poetic language. Mystical experiences have the ironic trait of not being well described in words but releasing a flood of words.

One of the best-known examples of ineffability comes from Bill Wilson, founder of Alcoholics Anonymous. "Suddenly the room lit up with a great white light. I was caught up into an ecstasy which there are no words to describe" ("Pass It On" 1984, 368–77).

Naturally Occurring: I knew at the time that I could never describe it. I knew I could never fully bring it back. There were not even words to describe it. I would never be able to talk to other people about this because it was something I couldn't explain. (Miller and C'de Baca 2001, 75)

Psychedelically Mediated: To cease to "BE," as I understand it, was not frightening. It was safe and much greater than I have words for or understanding. Whatever is larger than the state of being is what was holding me. (629)

There's good reason that words are inadequate. We build and exercise our language in our ordinary default state of mind, so it is a tool of that state and doesn't transfer as well for other states. Imagine if you dreamed but few other people did. It would be difficult to describe a dream to nondreamers. Similarly, it's difficult to describe mystical experiences to someone who has never had one. Skills in our ordinary state may not transfer well to other states, and a vocabulary learned for one state may be less useful in others. On the other hand, as more people have mystical experiences—whether psychedelic-induced or via the many other routes—will it become increasingly easy to communicate? Knowing the names for the ingredients of mystical experience as this chapter describes them may make talking about these experiences easier.

Changes in Attitudes and Behavior
One of the best-known examples of nondrug changes in behavior is Bill Wilson's. His quotation above continues:

And then it burst upon me that I was a free man. Slowly the ecstasy subsided. I lay on the bed, but now for a time I was in another world, a new world of consciousness. All about me and through me there was a wonderful feeling of Presence, and I thought to myself, "So this is the God of the preachers!" A great peace stole over me and I thought, "No matter how wrong things seem to be, they are right. Things are all right with God and His world." ("Pass It On" 1984, 368–77)

The sense of awe and a permanent shift in perception are normal—but not uniform—results of mystical experiences. For Wilson the experience of hitting bottom and rebounding to a mystical experience changed his mind and cured his alcoholism. In the 1960s and 1970s psychedelic mystical experiences were investigated as treatments for addictions, including alcoholism. Today, leads from those times are being unearthed and reexamined. Psychedelic treatments do not follow the standard medical path of relying on the direct biological effects of drugs on the body. Psychedelics produce—sometimes and under the right conditions—mystical experiences, and, as with Bill Wilson, it is these experiences and integrating them into one's life that cure.

The same experiences often have an impact that extends beyond curing to caring for others.

Naturally Occurring: Sometimes there is a newly experienced sadness and compassion for the amount of suffering in the world, and a positive desire to take part in alleviating it. (Miller and C'de Baca 2001, 15)

Psychedelically Mediated: The understanding that in the eyes of God—all people . . . were equally important and equally loved by God. I have had other transcendent experiences; however, this one was important because it reminded me that God is truly and unconditionally loving and present. (629)

The attitudes of equality and the desire to help others show up Bill Wilson's story again. It is especially relevant because he first had the nondrug, hitting-bottom mystical experience mentioned above; then on August 20, 1956, he had an LSD session under the direction of philosopher Gerald Heard and Dr. Sidney Cohen, one of the leading psychedelic experimental therapists of the 1960s. Bill had the following psychedelic mystical experience.

Bill was enthusiastic about his experience; he felt it helped him eliminate many barriers erected by the self, or ego, that stand in the way of one's direct experience of the cosmos and of God. He thought he might have found something that could make a big difference to the lives of many who still suffered. ("'Pass It On'" 1984, 371)

Change in behavior also presents an oddity in mystical experiences. Some people change their values, motivation, and behavior, but others treat their mystical episodes as strange interludes and go right back to being their old selves. Why? This is one of the big unanswered questions in mystical studies.

LINKED QUESTIONS

If mystical experiences—nonpsychedelic or psychedelic—alter everything, as Van Dusen said, there is no way to finish discussing them. With that in mind, here are some of my favorite related questions.

Life after Death, but Which Death?

Perhaps we are massively misinformed when we consider the spiritual meaning of "life after death." Which death? Body or ego? Feelings of being cared for, unity with a loving Great Other, forgiveness of oneself and others, increased understanding, charity toward others, timeless eternity, and feelings of rebirth into a new life after the experience—these characteristics of mystical experiences also appear in religious descriptions of postmortem heavenly rest. Because most people (including clergy, theologians, and religious philosophers) don't know firsthand about ego death, do they mistakenly think that death in religious texts means mortal, bodily death? If they could experience the ego-loss of mystical experiences, say during their professional training, would they (could they) reinterpret this fundamental religious belief? Even if they can't reinterpret, an experience of ego death might at least serve as a reasonable facsimile, a preparation, a guide toward physical death.

Is There a Connection with Birth?

Are there connections between mystical experiences, life in the womb, and other birth experiences? Might some of the power of mystical experiences come from tapping in to these earliest memories? It's helpful to know about Stanislav Grof's decades-long use of LSD in clinics and his map of the mind that comes from those efforts. In *LSD: Doorway to the Numinous,* Grof, the world's foremost researcher on the clinical effects of LSD psychotherapy, presents a four-level map of our minds—abstract and aesthetic, personal biography, perinatal, and transpersonal.

The perinatal level has to do with womb and birth experiences, and Grof notes strong similarities between the feelings engendered by mystical experience and by positive early life in the womb. Do mystical experiences tap in to this deep part of our minds? *LSD: Doorway to the Numinous* presents numerous parallels with undisturbed uterine life. Among them are an oceanic type of ecstasy and the experience of cosmic unity (2009, 104–5). Grof notes this parallel: "Observations from such sessions suggest that undisturbed intrauterine experiences are closely related to religious and mystical enlightenment" (112).

The sense of mystical union can take the form of a "Good Womb" experience. People feel a sense that all is right with the cosmos, that a powerful being is supplying all that is needed. One *Quantum Change* interviewee expressed the relaxed basking in goodness.

> I didn't really hear any voices or anything. It was more like they were trying to soothe me and comfort me and say, "Don't worry, just relax." It was kind of a soothing feeling, like when a mother holds a baby. (Miller and C'de Baca 2001, 82)

Just as positive womb experiences may provide a basis for mystical experiences, negative womb experiences may provide a basis for mental problems, often severe ones, but this is beyond the scope of this book, as this topic moves us into the psychotherapeutic uses of psychedelics.

The end of the birth process, the baby's emergence, presents other parallels with mystical experiences (Grof 2009, 104–5): the expansion of space and overcoming the limits of time and space, feelings of rebirth and redemption, humanitarian and charitable tendencies, and occasional grandiose feelings of success and triumph. Bill Wilson's sense of liberation during his nonpsychedelic mystical experience expressed this:

> Suddenly the room lit up with a great white light. I was caught up into an ecstasy which there are no words to describe. It seemed to me, in the mind's eye, that I was on a mountain and that a wind not of air but spirit was blowing. And then it burst upon me that I was a free man. ("'Pass It On,'" 1984, 370–71)

Can these connections between mystical experiences and the perinatal level be real, or are they merely coincidences? Some people object to the possibility of remembering these experiences because our brains at those early stages of development are not sufficiently developed to be able to remember in the usual cognitive sense. In a 1986 article "Taking Birth Trauma Seriously," pharmacist June Riedlinger and writer Tom Riedlinger examined Grof's perinatal ideas and proposed that "dedicated research by psychologists, psychiatrists, psychobiologists and medical scientists" be undertaken. With the founding of the Association for Pre- and Perinatal Psychology and Health, work now continues along these and parallel lines.

Do Mystical Experiences Provide a Clue to Rapid, Powerful Learning?

Everything we do entails using our brains. Whether we are learning how to recognize the difference between two sounds, thinking about something, practicing a skill, or reacting emotionally, our brains are active. But when we are learning to do any of these things, at first the neurons in our brains make weak, tentative contacts with other neurons. As we practice, the links between cells become stronger and eventually grow a circuit. This is what usually, but not always, takes place.

Sometimes this learning process happens quickly, almost in a flash. Repeated practice accounts for slow growth, but in traumatic experiences and mystical experiences pathways seem to be formed almost immediately. How? This rapid formation of brain circuits needs to be studied. Knowing how this happens will improve our knowledge of our brains, but more than this, it might be a clue to how to accelerate the usual, step-by-step learning process. Can we trigger such learning? Traumatizing people is not such a hot idea, to say nothing of the difficulty of obtaining the approval of an institutional review board. The obvious answer, of course, is providing peak or mystical experiences as a model.

A second fascinating related question about establishing brain circuits occurs. When a neuronal circuit is established, every additional time it is used it becomes stronger and more easily activated by future events. Analogically, at each use a hiking path gets worn down, making it easier to be traversed. Does this apply to mystical experiences? Will a psychedelic-induced mystical experience establish a path? Will that path make it easier for later events in the person's life to trigger other mystical experiences? Will several experiences strengthen the neural path into an easily followed one? In short, do mystical experiences beget mystical experiences?

Are Mystical Experiences What Maslow Called "Peak Experiences"?

In 1956 psychologist Abraham Maslow presented "Cognition of Being in the Peak Experience" as his presidential address to the Division of Personality and Social Psychology of the American Psychological Association (1962, 67–96). After identifying peak experiences as a trait of self-actualizers (surprising to him at first), he pointed to missing information in psychology—"[S]o far as I know [peak-experiences] have never received the attention of psychologists or psychiatrists"—and he ended his lecture by challenging his colleagues to study this aspect of healthy functioning scientifically. This was one root of transpersonal psychology.

Do peak experiences, as Maslow described them, qualify as mystical experiences? In his biography of Maslow, Edward Hoffman's summary of Maslow's description of these events sounds very similar to the POTT MUSIC ingredients of mystical experiences.

> Based on his phenomenological reports, these included temporary dislocation with respect to time and space, feelings of wonder and awe, great happiness, and a complete though momentary loss of fear and defense before the grandeur of the universe. People typically mentioned that polar opposites, like good and evil, free will and destiny, seemed transcended in such instances; everything in the cosmos was connected to everything else in a unity of splendor. (Hoffman 1988, 226)

While there are overlapping elements, the fit between peak experiences and mystical experiences is not perfect. In their chapter on mysticism from the *Psychology of Religion,* Hood, Spilka, Hunsberger, and Gorsuch—all professors of psychology—call peak experiences "a concept loosely related to, but perhaps broader than, mystical experience" (1996, 241). They write with some authority, as three of them are past presidents of the Psychology of Religion Division of the American Psychological Association, and all four are recipients of the division's William James Award.

Unrecognized by most psychologists, late in his career Maslow revised his famous needs hierarchy (see figure 2.1) and linked the new model to mystical experiences. Self-transcendence superseded self-actualization at the top.

> I should say that I consider humanistic, third force psychology to be transitional, a preparation for a still "higher" fourth psychology, transpersonal, transhuman, centered in the cosmos rather than in human needs and interest, going beyond humanness, identity, self-actualization and the like. (Maslow 1962, iii–iv)

Maslow extended the link to mystical experiences in "Theory Z," published in the *Journal of Transpersonal Psychology* in 1969, where he described the differences between two degrees of self-actualizing people,

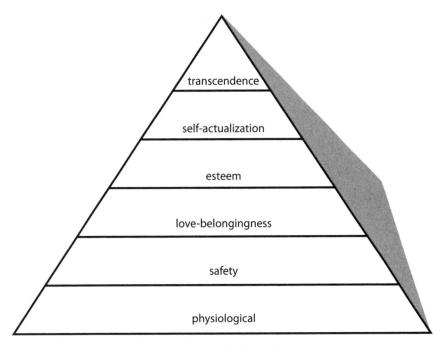

Figure 2.1. Maslow's Needs Hierarchy

"those who were clearly healthy, but with little or no experience of transcendence, and those in whom transcendent experiencing was important and even central" (31). The "transcenders" manifest several of the characteristics of mystical experiences including times of unitive consciousness, mystic, sacral, or ecstatic states, and cognitions that changed their perception of themselves and the world. This is yet another citing of the cluster of ingredients that compose a mystical experience.

Maslow went on to cofound the field of transpersonal psychology. The study of mystical experiences—both psychedelic and nonpsychedelic—is a central topic in this field of psychology (Roberts and Winkelman 2013). Maslow's challenge from half a century ago to include peak experiences is being met by the nonpsychedelic work of Miller and C'de Baca in *Quantum Change,* the psilocybin experimentation of the Johns Hopkins team, Ralph Hood's *Mysticism Scale,* and transpersonal theoretical writings. Thanks to psychedelics, experimental studies are now being added to phenomenological reports and clinical cases. The peak experience trail that was largely deserted in the late twentieth century is being paved and widened in the twenty-first: scientific and scholarly traffic is increasing steadily.

SUMMARY

What are some of the alterations that these all-altering experiences bring about? What accounts for them? Are the specific nine ingredients of mystical experiences merely the surface appearance of a more fundamental transformation that undergirds wider changes? Yes. As Miller and C'de Baca observe, the mystical-type quantum change "leaves behind a permanent shift in perception" (2001, 89). Below this is a different sense of self, of what it means to be a person. How that shift shows up in a person's life is the subject of the next few chapters.

3

Raising Values

A handy image for understanding how psychedelics raise values is to imagine a colonial-style lantern with its four sides made of transparent glass. Inside the lantern a candle is burning, but the four glass sides are covered with dirt, mud, or other gunk. The candle is our inner, spiritual nature, our better human nature, and its values. The dirt on the glass sides is our ego and its addictive desires, especially for money, fame, and power. To let the light shine through, we need to clean off the glass. Mystical experiences do this by transforming values, replacing low, self-centered values with higher ones.

The exploration of several lines of evidence gathered independently by people working separately reveals their corroboration, resulting in conclusions that are stronger than those that come from a group of like-minded people from one field working together. One of the significant shared conclusions in this field is that when mystical experiences provide ego transcendence and a sense of unity with others, then motivations and values shift from those that are self-centered to those that center more on a group, society, humanity, and even the cosmos. People who have had mystical experiences see their responsibilities, actions, and inactions in a wider context.

The line of reasoning here is quite straightforward: experiences affect people's values. Mystical experiences provide feelings and thoughts of identifying with all humanity, feeling safe and at home in the world, forgiveness and charity to oneself and to others, and especially a decrease in self-centeredness with its attendant values of the "seven deadly sins." The path of change can be diagramed as shown in figure 3.1.

Moral Development: The Mystical Path

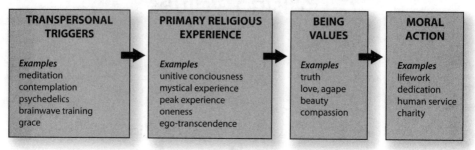

TRANSPERSONAL TRIGGERS	PRIMARY RELIGIOUS EXPERIENCE	BEING VALUES	MORAL ACTION
Examples meditation contemplation psychedelics brainwave training grace	*Examples* unitive conciousness mystical experience peak experience oneness ego-transcendence	*Examples* truth love, agape beauty compassion	*Examples* lifework dedication human service charity

Figure 3.1. Moral development: the mystical path

A statement that epitomizes this type of change is found in James Fadiman's 1965 dissertation at Stanford, Behavior Change Following Psychedelic (LSD) Therapy. During a "Behavior Change Interview," one person expressed his newfound dissatisfaction with I-ness and its values. "Money, power, prestige—Yale conditioning. It has not been erased from my mind, but a big chunk has been erased; perhaps now it is in proper perspective" (111). His 2011 book, *The Psychedelic Explorer's Guide,* presents this and other information in a reader-friendly format.

However, like other results of mystical experiences—particularly psychedelic ones—this shift is in the "sometimes" and "maybe" category, not something that always happens. The questions of how often and why some people make this shift and others do not is a topic that needs more research. Even more important, do mystical experiences represent a path of moral development? Or perhaps mystical experiences are a way of connecting people to values learned earlier in life. These are fundamental questions about where our values come from and deserve extensive attention.

THE ROOT OF VALUE PROBLEMS
I—A Case of Mistaken Identity

Where does the egoic gunk on our lantern's sides come from? A handy way to understand it is the seven deadly sins as they appear in literature. The leader of the Mud and Gunk Gang is Pride. The word *pride* in this context means excessive self-absorption, egocentrism, always wondering what's-in-it-for-me? Inflated ego is another way to say it. A realistic and efficient ego is a helpful servant that we need to function in daily life, but when it dominates us, it is a destructive and addiction-generating boss. Pride's six henchmen try to satisfy Pride's self-centered focus: Envy, Anger, Laziness, Greed, Lust, and Gluttony. Gluttony often includes drunkenness, but sometimes Booze gets personified on his own.

There is wise psychological insight in these portraits. These characters are the values of self-centeredness, but imagining them as if they were separate characters allows us to examine them as if they were outside ourselves: actually they are our own inner traits. They are the personal gunk that keeps us from letting the higher light through the lantern glass. They hide our deeper transpersonal motivations inside. Now research is showing that one way to rid ourselves from the domination of these self-centered demons is to wash them off the panes of glass with mystical experiences.

Greed, Money Addiction—More Is Never Enough

The more the seven deadly sins try to satisfy Pride's endless desires, the more Pride wants; this is addiction. America's major current addiction is to money. The American Psychiatric Association and the World Health Organization list nine criteria for drug dependence (Perrine 1996, 4). Substituting *money* for *drugs* shows how easily they describe money addicts as well.

- Taking pleasure in money more often or in larger amounts than needed
- Unsuccessful attempts to quit, persistent desire, craving
- Excessive time spent in money seeking

- Feeling intoxicated at inappropriate times, or feeling withdrawal symptoms from money at such times
- Giving up other things for money
- Continued use/spending, despite knowledge of harm to oneself and others
- Marked tolerance in which the amount needed to satisfy increases at first before leveling off
- Characteristic withdrawal symptoms from money or its substitutes
- Thinking about money and ownership to relieve depression or other unpleasant emotions

While we need money to meet our daily needs, the behaviors that satisfy those needs can become exaggerated and take over. Money addiction is detached from our real needs and begins to exist on its own, even taking over our lives. Because Pride's needs are never filled, money becomes a desire on its own, and there is always a desire for more. How can you tell if you are a money addict? According to the American Psychological Association and the World Health Organization, if you meet three of the nine criteria above, you qualify as *mildly* addicted. If you meet five, you are *moderately* addicted. If you meet seven, you are *strongly* addicted.

The parallel between money addiction and drug addiction is more than a mere analogy. According to *Your Money and Your Brain,* a 2007 book by Jason Zweig, who edits *The Intelligent Investor,* the brain chemical dopamine (how aptly named!), the other neurotransmitters, and the parts of our brains that respond to money, and even to the expectation of money are the same ones that light up when people expect addictive drugs and actually take them. Money addiction is physiologically real.

Lower Games vs. Higher Games

Robert S. de Ropp presents our inner battle between lower level values and higher ones in terms of selecting our life's purpose. De Ropp, a research biochemist who became interested in the effects of drugs on the human mind, divides life goals—"games," as he calls them—into two major groups. In his book 1968 *The Master Game* he lists the lower games: glory and victory, fame, and wealth. These are the lower I-me-mine pride-centered motivations. He calls them "object" games. The higher games—"metagames"—are beauty, knowledge, salvation, and awakening. They typically become stronger after mystical experiences. *Pathways to Higher Consciousness Beyond the Drug Experience* is de Ropp's subtitle; it nicely expresses the idea that it is not a drug experience itself that counts most, but what happens afterward, how the ingredients of a mystical experience affect one's life. The self-transcendence that at times results from mystical experiences dethrones Pride, or at least sets the self aside temporarily.

OSTENTATION NATION

Why are we stuck with so many low-level values? Consider that our yearnings for lower values such as glory, fame, and wealth are never satisfied and, more importantly, never can be satisfied. For this reason, they lead to a driven and treadmill life: haunting ambitions, competitive drives, a constant need to prove oneself. This sounds like the summary of watching a night of TV, doesn't it? There are few TV shows or movies that do not approvingly promote these values. Sometimes they show people being driven to violence or going crazy trying to satisfy these unsatisfiable drives. Many, probably most, of our day-to-day heroes and heroines are addicts trying to prove themselves, buy things, impress others, or are otherwise slaves to the Mud and Gunk Gang.

By appealing to Greed, Envy, Gluttony, Lust, Anger, and Laziness, ads are virtually all about Pride-satisfying consumption. "Buy this and you'll be happy." "Buy more and you'll be happier." Gluttony, by the way, is not restricted to food and drink. It includes consumption (ownership) in general. Is it any wonder we are a nation of fat people, driving fat cars, living in fat houses with overstuffed closets?

Jesus's $7,100 Wristwatch and the Moral Economy
QUIZ: If Jesus or any other religious leader were alive today and given $7,100, which of the following would he not do?

A. Buy a $7,100 wristwatch (a.k.a. chronograph)
B. Find a home for a homeless person
C. Buy clothes for an unemployed person
D. Provide water for the shantytown poor

This quiz points out three mutually supporting economic ethical levels. The first is internal: a person is so single-focused on his or her ego that the transcendent part, the candle within, is blocked. Buying more junk = more moral gunk. Second: even if someone has enough money to lavish on self-decoration and self-aggrandizement, the ethical question posits, "Is this the most moral use of that money?" A $6,725 ring (as advertised on Feb. 9, 2011, apparently with Valentine's Day in mind) could buy 672 mosquito nets to save lives of people in malaria zones. The $8,835 wasted on another chronograph could buy 73 sheep for peasant families in Peru or as many pigs for a family in Cameroon or 4,417 starter flocks of ducks and geese at $20 each to provide protein nourishment and a way of earning money for the impoverished around the world (Heifer International 2011).

Actually, $7,100 for a wristwatch is a poor-man's ostentation. For $28,218 one can buy a Hublot limited-edition carbon-fiber King Power Abu Dhabi chronograph (Hublot 2012). Apparently, this is a bargain price too. The May 11, 2012, online issue of *How to Spend It,* a supplement of the weekend *Financial Times,* lists the price at £25,600, approximately $38,400. Do the people who buy such morally sleazy things ever consider what suffering might be relieved with this money or how many lives might be saved?

Every purchase is three moral decisions:

Individual Budget: Do I have the money to pay for it?
Social-Economic: Would my money be better spent relieving suffering, say, or by providing a job for an unemployed person?
Spiritual Economy: Is this purchase just more mud and gunk obscuring the glass of my higher-values lantern?

A Cultural Craziness

Thanks to advertising, there is no end of places to observe how Pride and his Mud and Gunk cronies come to dominate our individual lives and national goals. Every day I check my daily update of examples of mad consumption-driven gluttony—maybe it should be called "lust for owning"—on pages 2 and 3 of the *New York Times*. The Sunday *Styles* section is even better. Vainglory, another of Pride's names, celebrates there daily. In contrast to the ads, the page 2 news index, "Inside the Times," summarizes the day's news, including a great many news items that have to do with people suffering. Next to a news item about starvation might be an ad for a diamond ring for $6,725. Next to an article about people in Africa who live on less than $2 a day is an ad for goofy-looking strappy shoes (price not listed). To me these shoes look like comic costume props from an *I Love Lucy* show, or perhaps part of a clown outfit. Raising the shoe immorality stakes even further, an ad in the August 31, 2011, issue offered "pearl embroidered pumps" for $1,450.

Greed and gluttony not only separate us from higher values but also can hurt innocent others, causing "economic collateral damage," when money is not used to relieve suffering. My all-time favorite example occurred in the *Times* on Friday, September, 17, 2010. On the front page above the fold an article with a picture tells the plight of itinerant poor living in a shantytown in Romania, where "the only source of water is a train station more than a mile away." Another front page article takes the poverty theme to the United States: "Recession Raises U.S. Poverty Rate to a 15-Year High." It is continued on page 3 with the caption of a picture of a man "who is homeless, looks for used clothing yesterday at Sacred Heart Community Center in San Jose, Calif." Ironically, the ads on pages 2 and 3 typically feature vainglorious ways to decorate oneself, oblivious to the fact that encouraging such consumption may be contributing to the news items. For example, that day, next to the article about poverty, are two ads for high-fashion handbags and ads for other luxury items. On the facing page is an ad for a wristwatch for $5,700.

Treatment: Identification with Humanity

Sometimes one of the effects of identifying with humanity and dropping the ego and its Mud-and-Gunk motivations during mystical experiences is concern for others and taking one's responsible place in the American family and in the human family. From that perspective the cost of a batch of bangles, say, at $435 is not the dollars spent but the improved life that is foregone. For someone with post-mystical insights, seeing show-off jewelry, show-off houses, show-off cars, show-off clothes, and other conspicuous consumption raises the question, "How many lives did that (jewelry, car, house, dress, and so on) cost? How much suffering might have been alleviated?" "At $250 each, how many harelips could have been mended?" (Smile Train 2011). From this perspective, so-called glitterati and fashionistas appear like death squads, not because their actions intentionally cause death and needless suffering but because lives could be saved and suffering reduced if resources were used ethically instead of misused to gratify Pride.

The Ego Has Problems: The Ego Is a Problem

The fault lies not only with a consumption-addicted society. There is an underlying intellectual reason that transitioning from lower values to higher ones is not as common as it should be. Most Western psychology and psychotherapy is ego centered, focusing on the individual person and why and how he or she becomes who he or she is. This dismisses the transpersonal aspect of human existence. Our lantern analogy focuses on the lantern's glass, not its inner candle. Likewise, Western clinical psychology helps someone overcome his or her problems and grow into a fuller person. A well-functioning person needs a healthy ego, but a full life depends on transpersonal experiences, which go beyond the ego.

For people who are stuck in self-centeredness, attachment to their egos is a problem. It keeps them from growing. The ego acts like an anchor. The experience of ego transcendence, whether from psychedelics or otherwise, lets people experience ego-transcendent values and motivations. Mystical experiences can weaken the ego's dominance and allow us to use it realistically as a tool, not let it use us as a master.

VALUE SHIFTS FROM NONPSYCHEDELIC MYSTICAL EXPERIENCES

What would it be like to live in a world where people were more caring about their families, communities, countries, the global human family, and the environment? Can mystical experiences move us toward this goal? Do they raise human values? Do they provide another path to moral development? Do both psychedelic mystical experiences and non-psychedelic ones raise ethical values? The answer to these questions is a strong "yes," but a tempered "yes," qualified by "sometimes, it depends, under the right conditions, for some people." What is the evidence this happens? How can we understand this shift? What are the implications for mind and society?

Studies in mystical experiences, the psychology of religion, and collections of anecdotes such as those in *Quantum Change* (Miller and C'de Baca 2001) report strengthened caring for others, increased compassion, forgiveness of others (and oneself), reduced resentment, acting to decrease suffering, and viewing one's actions in a wider context that includes society, humanity, and even the whole cosmos. The authors of *Quantum Change* noted the common theme of caring for others this way, "Sometimes there is a newly experienced sadness and compassion for the amount of suffering in the world, and a positive desire to take part in alleviating it" (15).

Having reviewed many studies and historical records, David Wulff, a professor of psychology at Wheaton College in Norton, Massachusetts, wrote in *Psychology of Religion*:

Among the predictable characteristics of mystical experience are a sense of sacredness of all life and a desire to establish a new, more harmonious relationship with nature and with other human beings. There is a corresponding renunciation of the various forms of self-seeking, including the ethos of manipulation and control. (1991, 639)

In keeping with Wulff's summary, in *Quantum Change* Miller and C'de Baca report particular changes that provide some details that augment Wulff's general finding. They asked their interviewees, "What was different after your experience?" The typical response was, "Everything." Expressing the all-things-are-altered theme, one person said, "Reality is the same. Life is the same. It's how I look at things and how things are pointed out to me that has changed" (2001, 127). Miller and C'de Baca found a profound realignment away from self-centered values when they asked their interviewees to compare their values before and after their mystical experiences using a list of fifty values. Here is how another of their quantum changers phrased it:

My motivations and my whole sense of direction in life have changed. My values changed. What I thought was important changed. I just completely shifted gears. It's given me a sense of purpose and direction I never had before, a real meaningful purpose in life. (130)

The table on page 47 shows how men and women ranked their most highly valued personal characteristics before and after a mystical experience (131).

Of course, such a shift in core values does not happen 100 percent of the time. Some people see their mystical experiences simply as strange interludes, and they go back to being their previous selves. Others reorganize their priorities and motivations. Why this is so is a fascinating unanswered question. In order not to overinterpret this shift, it is important to remember that Miller and C'de Baca were not in a position to ask their interviewees to order their values before their mystical experiences and then again afterward. The "Before" lists came from their interviewees looking backward to recall their pre-experience values after they had their mystical experiences.

THE MOMENT THAT TURNS YOUR VALUES UPSIDE DOWN

(Most Highly Valued Personal Characteristics
Before and After a Mystical Experience)

MEN		WOMEN	
Before	**After**	**Before**	**After**
Wealth	Spirituality	Family	Growth
Adventure	Personal Peace	Independence	Self-esteem
Achievement	Family	Career	Spirituality
Pleasure	God's Will	Fitting In	Happiness
Be Respected	Honesty	Attractiveness	Generosity
Family	Growth	Knowledge	Personal Peace
Fun	Humility	Self-control	Honesty
Self-esteem	Faithfulness	Be Loved	Forgiveness
Freedom	Forgiveness	Happiness	Health
Attractiveness	Self-esteem	Health	Creativity
Popularity	Loving	Faithfulness	Loving
Power	Intimacy	Safety	Family

VALUE SHIFTS FROM PSYCHEDELIC-BASED MYSTICAL EXPERIENCES

Reports of value shifts after psychedelic mystical experiences run parallel with those from nonpsychedelic ones. Wulff's summary of values enhanced by nonpsychedelic mystical experience—sacredness, harmonious relations with humans, caring for the environment—are paralleled by elements mentioned in the closing paragraphs of Grof and Bennett's *The Holotropic Mind,* as arising from "responsible work with nonordinary states of consciousness."

As their level of aggression decreased, they became more peaceful, more comfortable with themselves, and more tolerant of others.

Their ability to enjoy life, particularly the simple pleasures of everyday existence, increased considerably.

Deep reverence for life and ecological awareness are among the most frequent consequences of the psychospiritual transformation that accompanies responsible work with non-ordinary states of consciousness. The same has been true for spiritual emergence of a mystical nature that is based on personal experience. (1992, 221)

The general change of values summarized by Wulff and Grof is composed of many specific changes, both of discarding lower values and adopting higher ones. Underlying most of these changes is the ego-transcendent ingredient. When the self is experienced as a psychologically wider person, existing in broader social contexts, as not separate from others, from the world, from the cosmos, or from God, self-centeredness dissolves and with it self-centered motivations and values.

Mystical experiences empower our nonegoic values such as spirituality, compassion, altruism, and openness. What is most important is not psychedelics or any other specific way of producing mystical experiences, but rather the experience itself; psychedelics are just one among many psychotechnologies of transcendence.

Just as Wulff spotted decreased self-seeking as a common trait of nonpsychedelic mystical experiences, Grof found a similar pattern with psychedelic experiences. "In this context, a driven and hectic life pattern, haunting ambitions, competitive drives, a need to prove oneself, and the inability to enjoy are seen as unnecessary nightmares from which one can awaken." The transcendent ingredient of mystical experiences appears again, "Following ego-death . . . excitement about the process of life replaces the compulsion to pursue the achievement of goals" (1985, 49).

Altruism

One person who had a spontaneous mystical experience described feeling this way to Miller and C'de Baca: "After that experience I became a different person. I became a more loving, kind, compassionate person.

It was like I hit on some part of me that was this good person. I hadn't been a bad person before, but I just hadn't been aware of the goodness and kindness in me." Why would a mystical experience bring about this cherished bit of self-discovery? When transcendence reduces self-centeredness, when unity helps us feel oneness with other people and groups and even all humanity, when these combine with a sense of blessedness and agapé, the result is loving-kindness, compassion, a desire to be active in service to others and to help all humanity and the world.

Wulff described it as "a more harmonious relationship with nature and with other human beings" (1991). "Deep reverence for life and ecological awareness," Grof called it. When sacredness is added, theists feel it is the sacred duty of the social gospel to do God's work by helping others and promoting justice. Atheists may feel a basic humaneness and joy in decreasing others' suffering.

Other sources spot this typical altruistic change that follows mystical experiences too. Perceiving humans as deeply interrelated and part of a larger whole increases the sense of compassion. At the same time people become more alert to suffering and feel sadness about it. They also feel a desire to help alleviate it. "I felt very ashamed of many things I had done in my life." It is the nature of "turn-around" situations to start with a recognition of one's faults and errors, feeling sad, guilty, or depressed about them. This guilt is often followed by self-forgiveness, resulting in a sense of release, which can fuel altruistic behavior.

A statement by one of the volunteers in the Johns Hopkins psilocybin study shows how one person moved toward caring for others: "The understanding that in the eyes of God—all people . . . were all equally important and equally loved by God" (Griffiths et al. 2008, 629). If a large number of people thought this way, what might the widespread effects be?

This apparently altruistic feeling grew in most of the Hopkins hallucinogen-naive adults. Twenty-nine volunteers had one session with psilocybin and on another day a session with methylphenidate (Ritalin). Neither they nor their in-session monitors knew which drug they were receiving on a given day. To measure altruism two months after their sessions, a Persisting Effects Questionnaire asked the volunteers to rate how their experiences, of both Ritalin and psilocybin, matched the following eight statements (2012).

- You have become more sensitive to the needs of others.
- You now feel a greater need for service to others.
- You are more tolerant toward others.
- You have a more positive relationship with others.
- You now feel more love toward others.
- You have greater interpersonal perceptiveness (i.e., sensitivity).
- Your negative expression of anger (e.g., ridicule, outward expression of irritability toward others) has decreased.
- Your social concern/compassion has increased.

With the greatest possible score being 100 percent if every response had been "extreme," the Ritalin sessions scored 19 percent and the psilocybin sessions 44.5 percent. The probability of this happening just by chance is less than 1 in 10,000. The Hopkins' volunteers also rated the psilocybin sessions as significantly higher regarding positive attitudes about life and self and the production of positive behavioral effects. Both of these effects were as strong as the gain in altruism. From responses to a Persisting Effects Questionnaire fourteen months later, the researchers still found "positive changes in attitudes, mood, altruism, and other behavior" (630). The score on the altruism scale remained high: it actually rose 1 percent.

James Fadiman's *The Psychedelic Explorer's Guide* contains the most complete follow-up of psychedelic experiences on a broad range of topics, values among them. Responding to the question "How were you, or what were you left with, after the LSD experience?" the percentages of his group responding to the following value and attitude statements (among others) were:

85%—A greater understanding of the importance and meaning of human relationships.

78%—A sense of greater regard for the welfare and comfort of others.

88%—Increased reliance on my own values and judgment, less dependence on others' opinions. (Fadiman 2011, 299–300)

Contrary to the generally accepted wisdom of the times regarding material values, the men reported increased income, along with less caring about respect from others but more interest in finding new work. Women showed less interest in income but more in job satisfaction. Fadiman interprets this to show that income became less important while satisfying work became more important. Why does this happen? In *Beyond the Brain,* Grof answers, "Following ego-death, the ability to enjoy life typically increases considerably. The past and the future appear to be relatively less important than the present moment, and excitement about the process of life replaces the compulsion to pursue the achievement of goals" (1985, 49).

Openness

After the age of thirty, personality usually does not change significantly, but in "Mystical Experiences Occasioned by the Hallucinogen Psilocybin Lead to Increases in the Personality Domain of Openness," a follow-up study of the Johns Hopkins psilocybin experiment, Katherine MacLean, Matthew Johnson, and Roland Griffiths, all at Johns Hopkins, found increased openness among volunteers who had mystical experiences (2011). Openness includes traits related to imagination, aesthetics, feelings, abstract ideas, and broadmindedness.

"Normally, if anything, openness tends to decrease as people get older," said Roland Griffiths, the team leader of the psilocybin study ("Single Dose" 2011), but 60 percent of the 51 participants had increased openness. The change occurred specifically among those who had a mystical experience. Because the participants reported themselves as regularly participating in spiritual activities (including both church and non-church activities such as meditation) and because more than half had postgraduate degrees, Griffiths cautioned against generalizing their results to the general population.

Transcenders' Values

Besides results arising from Wulff's studies on the psychology of religion, Grof's LSD therapy, de Ropp's metagames, Miller and C'de Baca's quantum changers, and the Johns Hopkins psilocybin experiments, another line of evidence converges from Abraham Maslow's study (1962, 1971) of people he considered the psychologically healthiest and most fully developed humans, a best-case sample. When studying self-actualizers, he unexpectedly found that people who experienced especially intense peak experiences—ones that would probably qualify as mystical experiences— seemed boosted a level beyond ordinary, nonpeaking self-actualizers.

As mentioned earlier, toward the end of his life Maslow revised his needs hierarchy by placing self-transcendence as a stage above self-actualization (Roberts 1978). Transcenders exhibit the standard features of mystical experience such as loss of self-consciousness, transcendence of time, existing in the present, and ego loss. Maslow also specifically mentions "mystic fusion" and a resulting value shift (1971). Typically mystic fusion can be "with another person or with the whole cosmos or with anything in between" (271). In *Toward a Psychology of Being* (1962), Maslow offers a list of the motivations and gratifications of self-actualizers. He called them "Being Cognition" (78). Here yet again is the cluster of values that appear in the ingredients in mystical experiences, in de Ropp's metagame players, in the *Quantum Change* interviewees, and in the volunteers in the Johns Hopkins studies:

wholeness	perfection	completion	justice	aliveness
richness	simplicity	beauty	goodness	uniqueness
effortlessness	playfulness	truth	self-sufficiency	

In "A Theory of Metamotivation," Maslow reported that when self-actualizers (probably including the higher-level self-transcenders) are asked about what they especially enjoy about their jobs, they are "apt to answer in terms of intrinsic values, of transpersonal, beyond-the-selfish, altruistic satisfactions, truth, rewarding of virtue and punishing evil"

(1971, 310). It is easy to imagine the *Quantum Change* people whose value shifts are shown in the table above as sharing these feelings such as the delight in bringing about justice, stopping cruelty and exploitation, loving the world as it is while trying to improve it.

Life Values, Empathy, and Coping

A two-country survey in 2006 both supports and challenges these observations in a different way. Michael Lyvers, a professor in the department of psychology at Bond University in Australia, and his colleague and teaching fellow Michael Lerner wondered whether the values and beliefs of psychedelic users were different from the values of people who used other illegal drugs and different from the values of social drinkers who did not use illegal drugs. In hopes of reducing cultural effects and to see whether the effects of psychedelic use transcended culture, they sampled 110 people in Israel and 73 in Australia. In "Values and Beliefs of Psychedelic Drug Users: A Cross Cultural Study" they looked at life values, empathy, and to what degree people felt that they were able to cope with stress. They investigated whether "life-changing experiences described as mystical or transcendental" are correlated with, or influence, values and beliefs (Lerner and Lyvers 2006, 143).

From the "Life Values Inventory," Lerner and Lyvers looked at nine values: spirituality, concern for environment, concern for others, financial prosperity, creativity, belonging, loyalty to family or group, achievement, and humility. Psychedelic users scored highest on spirituality, concern for others, and concern for the environment. On the "Emotional Empathic Tendency Scale," psychedelic users and users of other illegal drugs scored highest, and on the "Sense of Coherence Scale," psychedelic users and nonusers of illegal drugs scored highest.

Appropriately, Lerner and Lyvers warn against misinterpreting their findings. As they say, "A question that naturally arises from the present findings is whether the above characteristics of psychedelic drug users preceded psychedelic use or resulted from such use" (146). Psychedelics may appeal to people who already have these characteristics. The same might account for why other users select the drugs they do too. If so, this helps explain why users of one drug may misunderstand why users of other drugs have their preferences. For example, alcohol users who drink in order to relieve stress or forget problems may wrongly suppose that psychedelic users do so for the same reason. The intensification of feelings that psychedelics produce would increase drinkers' stress and possibly frighten them. This is probably an origin of some "bad trips." Another place this error shows up is when so-called drug experts suggest that people take psychedelics to escape reality. The experience is just the opposite; people who use psychedelics experience their use as intensifying reality, making it "realer than real," as we saw in the previous chapter.

SUMMARY

When a number of separate research paths lead to overlapping conclusions, the combined results are more credible than those from any one path alone. What generalization about values comes from studies of mystical experiences? Mystical experiences—both psychedelic and nonpsychedelic—raise people from a self-centered I-me-mine direction in their lives to higher motivations, concerned with being of service to others and to the earth, or even to cosmic responsibilities.

4

The New Religious Era

FROM RITUAL TO WORD
TO EXPERIENCE

This chapter offers three big ideas. The first is new: we are transitioning from word-based religion to experience-based religion, a change that may turn out to be as broad and as deep as the religious transformation five hundred years ago when text-based religion replaced the dominate rite-based religion. A graphic version of this idea is shown in figure 4.1.

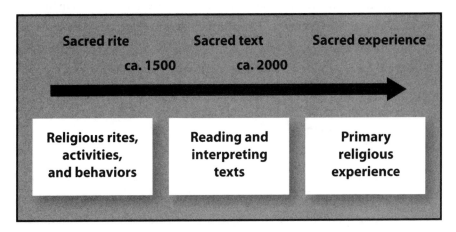

Figure 4.1. From rite to text to experience

The second and third ideas are not new but support the first. The second idea is that mystical experiences form a foundation of religion that gives rise to beliefs, rituals, ethics, and organizations. The third idea is that, under the right conditions, psychedelic plants and chemicals can—but do not always—produce mystical experiences.

Democratizing Text—Around the Year 1500

Around 1500, moveable type and the printing press democratized access to religious texts. The Reformation and the Counter-Reformation followed. General literacy and public education became important so that people could read religious texts. The growing importance of words nourished reason and science. While older religious observances of the prior period continued, new word-centered activities such as reading texts and interpreting them overlaid and overcame the older religion-as-rite era. New interpretations resulted; new churches flourished. Most important, text became an increasingly powerful source of religious ideas and a standard for judging them. Over time the locus of Western religious activity shifted from rites to reading, from observances to Bible, from participation to verbalization. In *The Case for God* religious writer and former nun Karen Armstrong marks the change this way:

> The success of the reformers was due in large part to the invention of the printing press, which not only helped to propagate this new idea but also changed people's relationship to text. . . . [A]nd this would make theology more verbose. . . . Ritual was downgraded. Instead of trying to get beyond language, Protestants would be encouraged to focus on the precise, original, and supposedly unchanging word of God in print. (2009, 171, 173)

We need only look at our current religions to see how accurate she is. In contrast to pre-1500, we approach religion verbally—through words. Texts, speaking, beliefs, sermons, catechisms, creeds, dogmas, doctrines, theology, and so on—all these are words. This overemphasis on words shows up today in the way we describe religions—as sets of wordy beliefs. To us, thoughts (cognitive processes) form religion. If we ask someone about his or her religion, we expect to hear about beliefs, not what rituals that person performs. The older rites certainly remain but lie obscured beneath a five-hundred-year-year blizzard of words.

Democratizing Primary Religious Experience—Around the Year 2000

Four questions and their respective answers point to a new stage of religious development that is unfolding: a transition from word-based religion to a new era of experience-based religion, one whose foundation is an intense, personal experience of the sacred.

1. *How would a direct primary spiritual experience affect someone?* A volunteer in the psilocybin study at the Johns Hopkins Medical Institute's Behavioral Pharmacology Research Unit answers this way: "The complete and utter loss of self . . . The sense of unity was awesome . . . I now truly do believe in God as an ultimate reality" (Griffiths et al. 2008, 629).

2. *If this happened regularly, how might wider society change?* Stanislav Grof, summarizing one of the effects of LSD psychotherapy, says: "Even hard-core materialists, positively oriented scientists, skeptics and cynics, and uncompromising atheists and antireligious crusaders such as Marxist philosophers suddenly became interested in a spiritual search after they confronted these levels in themselves" (Grof 1975, 97–8).

3. *What if religious studies programs, divinity schools, seminaries, religious orders, and similar religious educational institutions could teach their students to know this?* Psychotherapist Frances Vaughan, describing her own LSD-based experience, conducted when LSD was legal: "I understood why spiritual seekers were instructed to look within . . . My understanding of mystical teaching, both Eastern and Western, Hindu, Buddhist, Christian, and Sufi alike, took a quantum leap" (Vaughan 1983, 109).

4. *What if this happened fairly regularly?* Data from the

fourteen-month follow-up of the Johns Hopkins psilocybin study states that "33 percent of the volunteers rated the psilocybin experience as being the single most spiritually significant experience of his or her life, with an additional 38 percent rating it to be among the top five most spiritually significant experiences" (Griffiths et al. 2008, 621).

These things have happened, and in spite of a begrudging society, others like them are happening to thousands of people. They are not happening in churches or during religious services. At religious educational institutions they occur only extracurricularly, but in some scientific research laboratories they are occurring regularly, assisted by psychedelics. "What would be the impact if the reported positive behavior changes also turned out to be real?" asks Mark Kleiman rhetorically. He is professor of public policy at UCLA, a highly regarded specialist in drug policy, and author of *Against Excess: Drug Policy for Results* and *Drugs and Drug Policies: What Everyone Needs to Know*. He answers his rhetorical question:

We might witness, within a few years, the fulfillment of Moses's prayer: "Would that all my people were prophets!" People unafraid to die might act differently than the currently accepted norm. Just how much enlightenment can our current social order absorb? We may be on the road to find out. (Kleiman 2011)

Today entheogens—psychoactive plants and chemicals used in a spiritual context—democratize access to primary religious experience. Just as the 1500s word-based reformation evolved into today's religious, social, and political world, will today's experience-based reformation nourish its distinctive future?

Probably the best-known—and the least followed—example of progressing from words to experience comes from the ultimate Catholic wordsmith of all times, St. Thomas Aquinas. After writing thousands and thousands of words and building an army of concepts during his life, an "infused contemplation" convinced him that everything he had written, thought, and argued "was no better than straw or chaff," and he stopped writing on his unfinished book.

St. Thomas's view is widely echoed today. Among the voices is that of Frances Vaughan, author of books on psychology and past president of the Association for Transpersonal Psychology. In "A Question of Balance: Health and Psychology in New Religious Movements" (1987), she spots the failure of orthodox religious practices to provide genuine experiences of transcendence. Current religion would be much empowered if it could provide them.

Characterizing another modern turn away from words and toward experience, now-retired Harvard theologian Harvey Cox notes in *The Future of Faith* that many people "who want to distance themselves from the institutional or doctrinal demarcations of conventional religion, now refer to themselves as 'spiritual.'" He sees an emerging Age of the Spirit "in movements that accent spiritual experience," "pay scant attention to creeds," and show "resistance to ecclesiastical fetters" (2009, 10). This institutional transfiguration, he says, combines Pentecostal direct experience of the Divine with the discipleship of social justice. In many people's minds, biblical literacy and pentacostalism are lumped together, but, as Cox clearly distinguishes, "Fundamentalists are text-oriented literalists who insist that the inerrant Bible is the sole authority. Pentacostals, on the other hand, though they accept biblical authority, rely more on a direct experience of the Holy Spirit" (200). Although Pentecostalism and entheogen churches share the importance of direct spiritual experience, they would make strange bedfellows, for their experiences are arrived at via radically different methods. A "Psychedelic Pentecostal Church" would be a sight to behold.

Cautiously, Cox fails to mention his own peyote experience many years before, described in *Turning East: The Promise and Peril of the New Orientalism.*

What I felt was an Other moving toward me with a power of affirmation beyond anything I had ever imagined could exist. I was glad and grateful. No theory that what happened to me was "artificially induced" or psychotic or hallucinatory can erase its mark. "The bright morning stars are rising," as the old hymn puts it, "in my soul." (1977, 47–48)

Instead of citing entheogens as one contribution to the direct experience aspect of the Age of the Spirit, Cox neglects the extensive writings and numerous websites devoted to entheogens and does not even mention Huston Smith's *Cleansing the Doors of Perception* (2001). Instead he hides behind a question, "Might the capacity for awe be enhanced by a drug similar to the ones that enhance memory or alertness?" (Cox 2009, 24). Later Cox mentions a prayer: "Give us this day our daily faith, but deliver us from beliefs" (213) from Aldous Huxley's novel *Island* but fails to mention that in Huxley's novel daily faith arose from a fictional entheogen, "moksha." Psilocybin, ayahuasca, LSD, mescaline, and similar entheogens are today's real-life mokshas.

Entheogens

The term *entheogen* is used for psychedelics that are intentionally used spiritually, that is, they generate (*engen*) the experience of god (*theo*) within. *Entheogen* was listed in the *Oxford English Dictionary's* September 2007 release of new words: "entheogen. *noun.* a chemical substance, typically of plant origin, that is ingested to produce a non-ordinary state of consciousness for religious or spiritual purposes" (*Oxford English Dictionary* 2011).

Accompanying this entry was the following note: "This word, used to refer to a psychoactive substance employed for spiritual purposes, has an ancient Greek etymon, but is only attested from 1977. The word was apparently coined as an alternative to the words hallucinogen *n.* and psychedelic *n.*, which were strongly associated with recreational drug use. Notably, those words also have classical etymons (from Latin and Greek, respectively) but are attested only from the mid-20th century. While classical etymologies are now relatively rare in neologisms in the general vocabulary, they continue to be common in terms arising in scientific and medical circles."

Gutenberg and Entheogenic Reformations

Figurehead	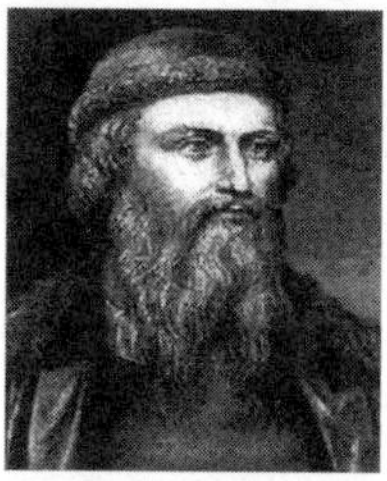	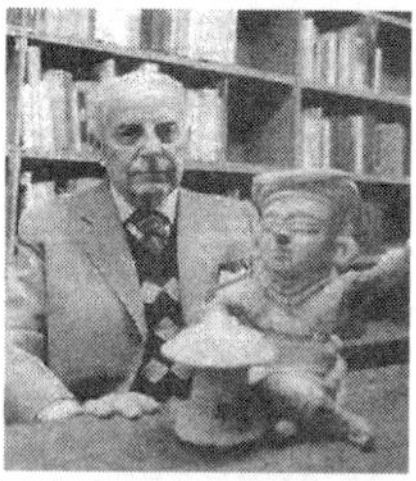
Icon	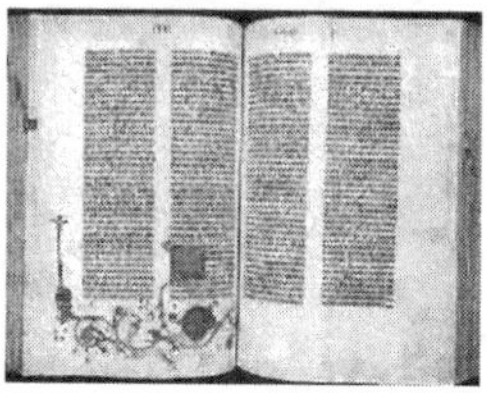	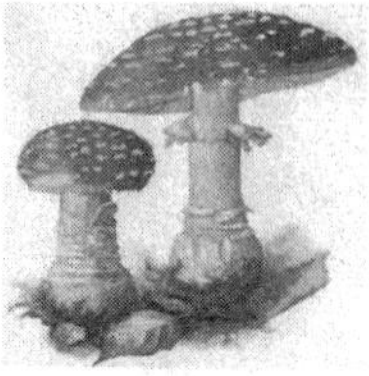
Democratized	Printed Word	Primary religious experience
Route to spiritual knowledge	Reading, study, thought (cognition)	Mystical experience (unitive conciousness)
Spiritual knowledge	Belief: doctrine, dogma, creed	Unmediated perception
Main academic disciplines	Theology and philosophy	Biology and psychology
Ethical action	Personal: Do and don't do to others	Transpersonal: Beyond self-interests
Education	Everyone should learn to read [the sacred texts]	People need to experience transcendence [everyone?]

Figure 4.2. The Gutenberg and entheogenic reformations

What do people who have had entheogenic mystical experiences think about them? Considering all the evidence in their 1979 review of the psychedelic literature, Lester Grinspoon and James Bakalar, then both on the staff of Harvard's Department of Psychiatry, summarize what they found: "It should not be necessary to supply more proof that psychedelic drugs produce experiences that those who undergo them regard as religious in the fullest sense" (Grinspoon and Bakalar 1979, 267).

MYSTICISM AS THE CORE OF RELIGION

The religious/spiritual effect of psychedelics often surprises people who use them for other purposes and unexpectedly stumble into the experience of intense sacredness, ego transcendence, and the other characteristics of mystical experiences. When this happened to me, I realized, "Religion really is about something"—it is about an experience people can have, not just a slow, millennia-old accretion of ideas, beliefs, habits, and rituals, not just a collection of supposedly historic events that may or may not have occurred as religious leaders currently describe them. My boyhood Connecticut Congregational church did not put much stock in mystical experiences. Surprised by my first unexpected mystical experience and subsequent ones, I wondered, "What is going on?" Exploring psychedelic writings soon led me to discover the extensive literature about states of unitive consciousness and the intricate complex of serious thoughts about them. Having since dedicated much of my personal life and professional efforts to researching them, it appears to me that this quest for meaningfulness is without end.

As I tentatively tried to understand my surprise mystical experience, one of my first discoveries was that mystical experiences—called by a legion of names—have been a central part of theology, philosophy, and religious practices throughout the history of religion. The centrality of mystical experiences is compactly stated in *Christianity and the World Religions.*

Indeed, isn't religion, above all—before it is doctrine and morality, rites and institutions—*religious experience.* Under the influence of Protestant theologian Friedrich Schleiermacher in nineteenth century Europe and philosopher-psychologist William James in early twentieth-century America, many Westerners have come out in support of the priority of religious experience. And isn't religious experience in its highest form *mystical experience,* as in India, where it seems more at home than anywhere else? (Kung, Ess, von Steitencron, and Bechert 1986, 168)

Until the late twentieth century, doctrine, rites, morality, and institutions were wrongly misunderstood as the basic elements of religion, and most people still see them as the building blocks of religion, rather than as secondary aspects whose roots grow in the soil of primary mystical experiences. In *Religions, Values, and Peak Experiences* psychologist Abraham Maslow wrote, "Most people lose or forget the subjectively religious experience, and redefine Religion as a set of habits, behaviors, dogmas, forms, which at the extreme becomes entirely legalistic and bureaucratic, conventional, empty, and in the truest meaning of the word, anti-religious" (1964). He also warned that mystical experiences are not all sweetness and light.

Focused on these wonderful subjective experiences, he may run the danger of turning away from the world and from other people in his search for triggers, *any* triggers. In a word, instead of being temporarily self absorbed and inwardly searching, he may become simply a selfish person, seeking his own personal salvation, trying to get into "heaven" even if other people can't . . . (viii)

Few people have experienced mystical oneness, so the twin errors continue, by which beliefs, rituals, ethics, and organizations are seen as the basic stuff of religion and the purpose of religion is seen as "getting into heaven." As more people experience primary religious experiences (PRE), the first error may diminish, but will the second one grow? For some mystics heaven is not a far-off place one goes to after death but a state of mind during mystical experiences, which one can experience during life.

Keeping the hopes and the dangers in mind, here is a graphic view of this chapter's second big idea.

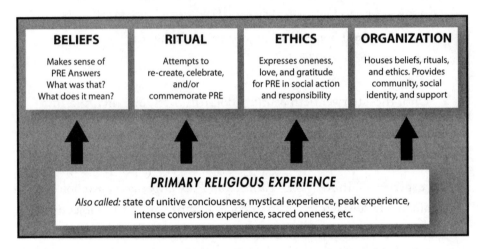

Figure 4.3. The taproot of religion—primary religious experience (PRE)— and its impacts

I want to be clear about what I am not saying. I am not saying that religion is nothing more than an attempt to understand, justify, or implement mystical experiences. Religion is more than the mystical inputs into religion, but those aspects are beyond the focus of this chapter.

CONTRIBUTIONS TO RELIGION FROM PSYCHEDELIC ENTHEOGENS

The entheogenic uses of psychedelics can allow people to explore the basement of religion, the primary spiritual experiences, that support its upper stories. We should not forget our wider culture's entheogenic uses of contemplative prayer, meditation, the martial arts, breathing techniques, yoga, and other ways. These and other spiritual psychotechnologies can also be paths to religion's foundations. Unfortunately, in this book we have room to describe only the psychedelic path to mystical experiences and have to leave the other paths for others to write about.

Specifically, entheogens have made noticeable contributions to beliefs, rituals, ethics, and organizations. As with any new, emerging field, some aspects are relatively well developed, while others are just beginning.

Contributions to Beliefs and Knowledge

The ideas that come from direct, personal sacred experience overlap but are not the same as those that come from reading about spirituality. In a manner of speaking, word-based religion is like reading a recipe, while mystical experience tastes the food. To put it another way, word-limited religion gives you a map to sacred blessedness or heaven; mystical experience takes you on a visit. To most people who are even moderately experienced with entheogens, concepts such as awe, sacredness, eternity, grace, agapé, transcendence, transfiguration, dark night of the soul, born-again, heaven, and hell are more than theological ideas; they are experiences.

Reactions to mystical experiences that affect beliefs come in three types. Some people may understand ideas that they previously had known of only verbally. Others do an about face, experiencing what is known as "conversion," and still others have their preconceptions strengthened and confirmed by their experiences.

Belief—Information

Frances Vaughan, Ph.D., former president of the Association for Transpersonal Psychology, author and coauthor of transpersonal books, and a psychotherapist in private practice, provides an excellent example of the breadth of knowledge that can come from a mystical experience in a prepared mind. Her insights illustrate five kinds of spiritual learning: philosophical theology, a widened interfaith scope, personal insight, spiritual practice, and psychological understanding.

The perennial philosophy and the esoteric teaching of all time suddenly made sense. I understood why spiritual seekers were instructed to look within, and the unconscious was revealed to me to be not just a useful concept, but an infinite reservoir of creative potential. I felt I had been afforded a glimpse into the nature of reality and the human potential within that reality, together with a direct experience of being myself, free of illusory identifications and constrictions of consciousness. My understanding of mystical teaching, both Eastern and Western, Hindu, Buddhist, Christian, and Sufi alike, took a quantum leap. I became aware of all great religions, and understood for the first time the meaning of ecstatic states. (Vaughan 1983, 109)

As Dr. Vaughan's statement shows, entheogens broaden understanding of religion beyond the confines of particular doctrines and creeds to a more inclusive perspective on spiritual development. After mystical experiences, particular religions, sets of beliefs, or rituals often become embedded in a wider perspective as one spiritual path among many. Rabbi Zalman Schachter-Shalomi sees psychedelics as reducing what he calls a "triumphant" attitude among clergy who see their own religion as the only good one, looking down on others (Schachter-Shalomi 2005, 195–205). He cites his daughter as expressing the desire for spiritual knowledge: "She asked, 'Abba! When you're asleep, you can wake up, right? But when you're awake, can you wake up even more?'" (196). People can, but do not always, experience this second awakening with entheogens.

Belief—Conversion

Conversion can be of more than one kind. In some cases it may be conversion to a specific religion. In others it may take the form of a conversion from an antispiritual view of human nature to a spiritual one, such as is shown by the passage about "hard-core materialists" from Grof's *LSD: Doorway to the Numinous* quoted earlier. More completely it reads:

In my experience, everyone who has reached these levels develops convincing insights into the utmost relevance of the spiritual dimensions in the universal scheme of things. Even hard-core materialists, positivistically oriented scientists, skeptics and cynics, and uncompromising atheists and antireligious crusaders such as Marxist philosophers suddenly became interested in a spiritual search after they confronted these levels in themselves. (2009, 97–98)

"These levels" he refers to are the perinatal levels of our minds, which are described more in chapter 11 of this book, "It's a Perinatal World." A more specific conversion account is described in *The Antipodes of the Mind* by Benny Shanon, professor of psychology at Hebrew University in Jerusalem, a highly respected cognitive psychologist and a veteran of at least 130 ayahuasca sessions. "Personally, if I were to pick one single effect of Ayahuasca that had the most important impact on my life . . . I would say that before my encounter with the brew I was an atheist . . . and when I returned back home after my long journey in South America, I no longer was one" (2002, 260).

Because a person's expectations, both conscious and unconscious, are a major input into psychedelic experiences, negative expectations as well as positive ones will often flavor a psychedelic session. In *The Hallelujah Revolution: The Rise of the New Christians,* British writer Ian Cotton reports on "Edward" and "Jill," young followers of a Christian sect. After taking an unidentified substance one evening, they suffered a traumatic and horrific session with Satanic feelings and thoughts. Their beliefs influenced their experiences. Later they felt forgiven, reborn, and Edward saw "a strip of water hanging in the air yet made of light and shimmering and it was at that moment I realized what had shot through me; it was the Holy Ghost" (1996, 127). Later that morning he said, "I saw this vision of the Cross" (128). He felt redeemed and forgiven by God. This demonstrates that negative expectations can be amplified and converted into both negative experiences and positive ones.

Sophie Burnham, a prize-winning author of books about angels, presents different experiences from others' writings. In *The Ecstatic Journey: The Transforming Power of Mystical Experience*, she names psychotechnologies for producing mystical experiences. "There are three ways of courting holy ecstasies: through age-old religious disciplines of prayer and fasting, the expression of the longing heart; through sacred dance and ritual; and last by ingesting intoxicants or hallucinogenic substances" (1997, 208–9). She reports on the positive experiences of several people who approached them with such a mindset. One of them said, "There was a Voice of Knowledge over to my left. It said *I am God*." She quotes W. T. Stace, who led the modern study of mystical experiences and, in turn, quoted one of his informants: "I had no doubt that I had seen God, that is, had seen all there is to see; yet it turned out to be the world that I looked at every day" (217).

World-renowned philosopher of religion Huston Smith, falls within the camp of people whose existing beliefs have been confirmed thanks to entheogens. Author of *The World's Religions,* the most adopted book in comparative religion courses, he believed in a theory of emanationism, but it was only as an idea until he took some mescaline at Timothy Leary's house on New Year's Day, 1961. He experienced his idea as a perception. "I was experiencing the metaphysical theory known as emanationism, in which, beginning with the clear, unbroken Light of the Void, that light then fractures into multiple forms and declines in intensity as it devolves through descending levels of reality" (Smith 2000, 11). Aware of the implications of this for theology and philosophy, he titled his essay "Empirical Metaphysics" and republished it as chapter 1 in *Cleaning the Doors of Perception.*

The experiences of Huston Smith, Edward and Jill, and Frances Vaughan are all instances of people's ideas seeming to become real in their perceptions. They moved from word-based beliefs to firsthand knowing confirmed during entheogenic experiences.

What are we to make of such portrayals? Have these individuals gained insights into how reality actually is? Or, do entheogenists merely uncritically confuse their beliefs with reality? Is the sense of objectivity (the "realer than real" feeling) misleading them, or is the noetic knowledge an insight into how things actually are? If a powerful sense of reality can be misleading during mystical states—when the reality rheostat is turned way up—on what grounds should we assume that our ordinary, default state's rheostat setting is accurate? Might some entheogenic insights be true and others untrue? How could we go about determining which is which? There are enough philosophical knots here to embroil at least one generation of philosophers, theologians, neurocognitive researchers, and other intellectually active people. Most important, thanks to entheogens it is now possible to surpass ordinary-state armchair philosophy and begin to study these topics with experiments.

A note of caution, however: no matter how ultimately true and certain an idea seems during a mystical experience, the sense of objectivity and noetic knowledge can be misleading. When the walls pulse or a smudge on a wall resembles a face during a psychedelic trip, most of the time people recognize that this is not really happening because it violates their sense of default-state reality. It is harder to be skeptical of one's abstract ideas when a sense of noetic truth adorns them. We should remember the possibly apocryphal story of William James's "Hogamous-Higamous" stumble, which contains some evolutionary behavioral truth and a nice dollop of humor but does not qualify as a major insight about the ultimate nature of the universe.

Contributions to Ritual

With the entheogenic reformation still in an early stage, the development of related rituals is also just unfolding. That process involves several difficulties. One arises from the problems associated with the meaningful transfer of rituals from one culture to another. Will rituals developed in the cultures of the upper Amazon work in North America, Europe, and elsewhere? Another issue is that mystical experiences are largely psychologically interior events, so group entheogenic services will necessarily have to allow inner introspection to occur. As with existing religious organizations, different personality types may feel more at home with particular types of service or ritual than another. For example, introverts may feel most at home alone or with one or two other people. Extraverts may enjoy group bonding amplified by entheogens. A third problem relates to the difficulty of arranging a service or ritual that would last as long as a drug effect lasts. A one-hour church service on Sundays is not going to do it. A fourth difficulty relates to the preparation of guides and determination of their capability (Jesse 2012). What qualifications do they need? Surely there are other questions. Leads for addressing these questions come from three sources: indigenous entheogen-using churches, accumulated knowledge from the 1960s to the present, and experimental protocols in current research.

Indigenous Rituals

According to Ralph Metzner, whose psychedelic interests stretch back to the 1960s at Harvard, where he was a graduate assistant for Timothy Leary and Richard Alpert, there is a "wealth of information in the anthropological literature on the indigenous use of sacred plants" (2002, 165). In "Ritual Approaches to Working with Sacred Plants," in Charles Grob's *Hallucinogens: A Reader,* he summarizes his observations of indigenous religious organizations in Africa, South America, and North America, identifying a list of common ritual elements: ceremonies held at night, moderate dosages, a format of circles, a ceremonial leader, a focus of attention such as an altar or fire, and prolonged rhythmic drumming, singing, or dancing (2002). As Metzner points out, the anthropological literature can provide leads, but probably not ceremonies that can be transferred item by item to contemporary American or European cultures.

Accumulated Knowledge

Some entheogenic ceremonies, however, have already been designed for the Western mind. Myron Stolaroff, who cofounded the International Foundation for Advanced Study in Menlo Park in 1961, is a grandfather of the design of psychedelic sessions. One of his books, *The Secret Chief*

Revealed, is a compilation of decades of his and Leo Zeff's (the "secret chief") reflections on the psychotherapeutic and entheogenic uses of psychedelics. At a small invitational conference on entheogens sponsored by the Council on Spiritual Practices and the Chicago Theological Seminary in 1995, he proposed "A Protocol for a Sacramental Service" (Stolaroff 2012).

Stolaroff points out that many people will not be at ease with entheogens, so in his "Protocol" he proposes three methods of socialization: 1) work with the person until he or she feels at ease about joining a group; 2) start with a less challenging entheogen such as MDMA; and 3) start with a low dose and work up to stronger ones (2012, 178–87). According to Stolaroff, for sessions to be successful, "Deep intention for a positive outcome can dissolve many barriers and resistances. Psychological health eases the passage" (180–81). Openness and the ability to surrender to experience are other pluses. The guide should be someone "who has a great deal of personal experience in using entheogens." The setting should be a comfortable room with ready access to natural beauty such as a garden.

Some psychotherapists like to use a "booster" dose if an original one does not produce the desired effect. A 2011 dose-response paper by the Johns Hopkins psilocybin team found, "Thus, it appears that having experience with lower doses facilitates the likelihood of having sustained positive effects after a high dose of psilocybin" (Griffiths et al. 2011, 663), thus confirming Stolaroff's approach of an ascending dose sequence. At the same time, however, "The acute anxiety/fear-producing effects . . . increased with increasing doses" (633). A therapist—whom Stolaroff believes introduced more than 3,000 subjects and more than 100 therapists to psychedelics—originally asked his clients to read spiritual literature, but he later decided that a better induction to the right attitude was a prayer by Francois de Salignac Fenelon, repeated twice.

Stolaroff's method combines therapy and spiritual development. From a transpersonal perspective the path of psychological growth followed far enough leads eventually to spiritual growth. As a step along this path, Stolaroff recommends meditation as a way of psychologically stabilizing a person. The entheogenic path, he implies, is not for everyone and, for many people, requires rethinking of religion. Church members and clergy are fond of thinking their denomination or sect is right for everyone, while few entheogenists would agree with such a perspective. For people who are not ready for entheogenic religion, psychedelic psychotherapy may be a good prerequisite.

In his 2011 *The Psychedelic Explorer's Guide,* James Fadiman addresses the how-to of rituals—both entheogenic and secular—drawing on his own experiences, his role as an assistant in Stolaroff's institute where legal sessions were conducted during the 1960s, and information accumulated in the decades since then. In part 1, on transcendent experiences, he makes it clear that the preparation of guides is paramount. Among the common issues for guides are their intentions, point of view, relationship with the voyager, social boundaries, transpersonal expression, and, appropriately, when to cancel or postpone. Later in the book he suggests structures and procedures for sessions intended for creative problem-solving and personal growth. As indicated by the subtitle—*Safe, Therapeutic, and Sacred Journeys*—his book goes far beyond the razzmatazz of common "I-dropped-acid" books to seriously reflect on how to ritualize the set, setting, and guidance to promote safe and productive psychedelic sessions.

In preparation for a 1995 conference on entheogens as sacraments, I started to prepare a bibliography of books, dissertations, and thematic issues of journals on this topic. I thought I would find a couple dozen books, perhaps as many as forty. However, as is testified to by the online archive that presents the results of that research, *Religion and Psychoactive Sacraments: An Entheogen Chrestomathy* (Roberts and Hruby 1995–2000), I found far more than anticipated. In 2000 I stopped the collection at 550 items in order to have time for my writing projects. The archive includes extended bibliographic information and selected excerpts from the publications but does not include articles, chapters, or websites and omits biological writings with specialized vocabulary that a nonspecialist would be unlikely to understand. The extensive anthropological writings were also given short shrift. If these things had all been included, the number of items would have run well into the thousands. Since the year 2000, about a hundred or more additional books and a small flock of dissertations would qualify too.

Experiment-Based Leads

Two other sources of clues to how entheogens might be used for spiritual development come from experimental studies that bookend the topic, the 1962 Good Friday experiment and its decades-later replication, the 2006 Johns Hopkins psilocybin study.

The classic example of experimental research using entheogens occurred in Marsh Chapel at Boston University on Good Friday 1962. Walter N. Pahnke, who was already a medical doctor and an ordained minister, conducted the most significant study to date on the entheogen-religion connection as the data for his doctoral dissertation in Religion and Society at Harvard Divinity School. He gave psilocybin (the active ingredient in psychedelic mushrooms) to ten graduate students from Andover-Newton Theological Seminary, while another ten received an active placebo. They met in a room-size chapel in the basement of Marsh Chapel at Boston University and listened to the upstairs service over a sound system. Pahnke wanted to know whether the psilocybin subjects would experience mystical states and whether they would do so more than the ten control subjects. They did, and what has become legendary in the psychedelic community as the "Good Friday experiment" remains a paradigmatic experiment. The test of concept was successful: the psilocybin subjects did report mystical experiences as measured by a scale derived from the 1961 work of W. T. Stace.*

This experiment may also be the most remarkable experiment ever in the social sciences. While the experiment of giving an entheogen to seminarians in a religious setting is unique, that is only one thing that sets the Good Friday experiment apart. In the social sciences,

_____

*Hood's *Mystical Experience Scale,* today's standard instrument in the field, grew out of the same source.

experimental studies are in short supply; this is even more so in religious studies. Those done outside controlled lab environments are scarce. Ex-lab experiments in which the subjects are administered a treatment only once are infrequent. Single treatment, ex-lab, experimental designs with measurable, long-lasting effects are rare, but in a twenty-five-year follow-up study of Pahnke's Good Friday subjects, Rick Doblin, Ph.D., founder and president of the Multidisciplinary Association for Psychedelic Studies, found:

> This long-term follow-up, conducted twenty-four to twenty-seven years after the original experiment, provides further support to the findings of the original experiment. All seven psilocybin subjects participating in the long-term follow-up, but none of the controls, still considered their original experience to have had genuinely mystical elements and to have made a uniquely invaluable contribution to their spiritual lives. (Doblin 1991, 73)

Having effects that persist twenty-five years from a single-treatment experimental study makes the Good Friday experiment remarkable enough, but there's more. What makes this experiment so amazing, Doblin reports, is that "the positive changes described by the psilocybin subjects at six months, which in some cases involved basic vocational and value choices and spiritual understandings, had persisted over time *and had deepened in some cases*" (73, emphasis added). An effect that is strengthened and deepened over a quarter of a century marks a permanent shift in the way the psilocybin subjects saw their world. Obtaining stable to increased results from a one-treatment experiment in a natural setting speaks to the power of entheogens as experimental treatments and more explicitly to the power of mystical experiences. Startling, powerful, original, unique, and persistent—these results certainly called for replications.

Finally, after forty-four years, they were replicated. By 2005 and 2006, however, research design, techniques, instrumentation, and statistical procedures had advanced several generations, and these advances brought research methods up to twenty-first-century standards. Thirty volunteers—cheers to the Johns Hopkins Psilocybin Team for calling them "volunteers" instead of "subjects" or "patients"—received psilocybin, but instead of twenty seminarians and their small group leaders meeting in one room, each volunteer took the psilocybin in a comfortable living room–like setting and was accompanied by two professional monitor-guides. They listened to a prerecorded CD of music, wore eyeshades to direct their attention inward, and relaxed on a couch. As with the Good Friday volunteers, each participant also took an active placebo, but at a different session, and neither the volunteers nor their monitors knew which drug was supplied in which session. The Baltimore study used more surveys to evaluate the effects of the session and even included Hood's Mysticism Scale.

The title of the first article on the study tells the results: "Psilocybin Can Occasion Mystical-type Experiences Having Substantial and Sustained Personal Meaning and Spiritual Significance" (Griffiths et al. 2006). The title of their follow-up study amplifies the first: "Mystical-type Experiences Occasioned by Psilocybin Mediate the Attribution of Personal Meaning and Spiritual Significance 14 Months Later" (Griffiths et al. 2008).

Their results give rise to two important questions.

Do entheogens provide secular rituals for spiritual development?
Does spiritual growth have to take place in religious organizations?

For more than half a century some psychedelicists have claimed that some—by no means all—of their experiences are spiritual. This idea is both vigorously supported and vigorously pooh-poohed. However, two-thirds of the Hopkins sample certainly thought their experiences were.

The successful results of the Hopkins study provide clues to how future religious rituals might be made successful too: selection and screening of participants is primary. They must be made to feel at ease with their monitors/leaders. As with psychedelic psychotherapy, they should be alerted to the range of what to expect, how they may feel, what they will do on their session day. Finally, it is best if they do not simply have an experience and go wandering off into the future; they should receive help as they make sense of their experiences and integrate them into their daily lives. As Roger Walsh points out in the next chapter, sustaining the experience is one of its most demanding aspects. In a few well-chosen words, Huston Smith directs our attention to the importance of mystical experiences, psychedelic or otherwise: "the goal, it cannot be stressed too often, is not religious experiences; it is the religious life" (1977, 155). There are two up-to-date sources on how to run sessions. Matthew Johnson, a member of the Hopkins psilocybin team, recommends procedures in his 2010 "Human Hallucinogen Research: Guidelines for Safety." A research procedure or protocol is, after all, a type of scientific ritual. James Fadiman gives directions for both guides and explorers in his 2011 *The Psychedelic Explorer's Guide*.

Contributions to Ethics

Chapter 3, "Raising Values," has largely covered the topic of ethics. However, several additional points need to be mentioned. One is that the movement toward more ethical action comes, in these cases, directly from the insights and feelings occurring during mystical experiences, not from written or spoken words, creeds, and so on. However, with general loving-kindness and social caring growing from the roots of mystical experiences, an embracing mystical attitude is likely to be in agreement with broad-based views of morality promoted by the churches (while disagreement on particular social mores is likely).

Antinomianism is the idea that one is above the law and can do as one wants. This is a problem—perhaps *danger* is a better word—with people who have mystical-type experiences from any source but do not transcend their egos fully, instead absorbing their experiences into their egos, making their egos stronger. They become more self-centered and self-inflated. While a sense of humbleness—"What did I do to deserve this wonderful experience? Why am I so lucky?"—is common, its opposite, ego inflation, can also result.

Contributions to Organizations

Looking at the current situation there is little to say about the possible contributions to organizations. The best-known use of entheogens is the use of peyote by the Native American Church. This has been supported by both the U.S. Congress and the Supreme Court (Smith and Snake 1996).

On the other hand, the situation for the ritual use of ayahuasca is unresolved and varies from country to country. The expansion of the Brazilian-founded Uniao do Vegetal Church and the Santo Daime Church into the United States and Europe exemplify the globalization of this new sacrament and raise as-yet unresolved issues over whether drug policy or freedom of religion should take precedence (Groisman and Dobkin de Rios 2007).

Brazil-based international ayahuasca scholar Beatriz Labate describes the growth of entheogenic organizations taking place following the growth of ayahuasca churches in South America and their spread to northern countries and especially the agreements between the Uniao do Vegetal and the U.S. Drug Enforcement Administration. She spots an "institutionalization project" consisting of bureaucratization of records, administrative organization, and establishing specialized leadership roles. Among other manifestations, these show up in forming a canon of spiritual teachings for the transmission of knowledge, more structured ritual processes, codification of lyrics and melodies, and the regulation of the processes of cultivating, obtaining, and cooking ayahuasca. The Amazonian UDV, she reports, "is creating a school that will teach courses to its members on growing and handling the species that constitute ayahuasca; the school will supply written curriculum and offer diplomas at completion" (2011, 3).

It remains to be seen whether established churches will catch on to the entheogenic reformation and begin to offer entheogenic mystical experiences in religious settings. Perhaps that would strengthen the beliefs of their congregants and even evangelize new members. Their current dedication—even idolatry—to "the word," however, keeps them anchored. To offer entheogenic sacraments, of course, specialized church leaders would have to be thoroughly prepared to provide psychological help if needed, as well as professional spiritual guidance. Just because someone is a member of the clergy, religious order, or other religious group, that does not qualify that person to be a guide.

Unfortunately, press accounts often underplay the series of professional cautions that go into laboratory research, or they may omit mentioning them altogether. A sentence from the Johns Hopkins 2011 study emphasized "it is important to recognize that the present study [and its precursors] was conducted in carefully screened volunteers who received ample preparation before sessions, were closely monitored during sessions, and had some continuing contact with study staff after sessions" (Griffiths et al. 664). Matthew Johnson's 2008 article "Human Hallucinogen Research: Guidelines for Safety" delineates the care that must be taken.

If Western churches do decide to offer entheogenic sacraments, such ceremonies might be best thought of as similar to religious retreats. A religious order or guild may want to develop the specialty of structuring, officiating, and running such retreats, for which they would need training in skills such as screening, preparing, and guiding participants during and after their experiences. I can imagine an order of nuns taking on this responsibility. At this point the clearest thing that can be said about how to plan and direct an entheogenic ritual is that it is a developing process, and more experience will yield clearer guidelines. For one thing, most experience so far comes from lab-based psychotherapeutic protocols (medical rituals), which are at odds with established personal experience.

Another caution for religious organizations that may want to develop religion in entheogenic directions is that such experiences are not for everyone. In the Good Friday experiment the participants were seminary students. Of course, their psychological set and the setting of a church would predispose them toward mystical experiences with sacred interpretations. In a second dose-response study, the Hopkins volunteers were carefully screened; only 18 people from 279 initial inquiries were included in the study (Griffiths et al. 2011, 650).

CONCLUSION

The word-based Reformation that took place five hundred years ago produced an earthquake swarm of schisms whose aftershocks continue today. As entheogens give us another step toward spiritual democracy, will the spread of direct, personal spiritual experience cause similar schisms in our future? It is likely that people will form new churches, one source of schism. As this happens there will also be enormous legal tangles to straighten out among human rights, freedom of religion, and drug policy. It is not at all clear who has the knowledge, experience, and perspective to make informed judgments on this topic.

> *Children of a future age,*
> *Reading this indignant page,*
> *Know that in a former time*
> *A path to God was thought a crime.*
> —AFTER WM. BLAKE

In their best uses, psychedelic mystical experiences should not just be a day's entertainment with no lasting benefits. Psychiatrist Roger Walsh is guest author of the next chapter, which analyzes the "sustainability problem." Weaving together medicine, philosophy, and shamanism, Dr. Walsh describes the importance of integrating these experiences into our daily lives, making them more than just another freaky Saturday.

5

Psychedelics and Religious Experiences

WHAT IS THE RELATIONSHIP?

ROGER N. WALSH, M.D., PH.D., D.H.L.

Roger Walsh, M.D., Ph.D., D.H.L., is a professor of psychiatry at the University of California Medical School at Irvine and also holds positions in the departments of philosophy and anthropology. This chapter draws on his 2003 article "Entheogens: True or False?" and 2007 book *The World of Shamanism*.

Q

The use of drugs to induce sacred states of consciousness has flourished throughout human history. Historical examples include the Zoroastrian *haoma,* the Australian Aboriginals' *pituri,* Zen's tea, and Hinduism's *soma,* otherwise known as "the food of the gods." In ancient Greece, *kykeon* inspired the Eleusinian mysteries and wine the Dionysian ecstasies.

However, in the modern West, psychedelics were all but unknown, until they crashed into a culture utterly unprepared for any of them in the 1960s. For the first time in its history a significant portion of Western society experienced powerful ASCs (altered states of consciousness).

Some of these states were clearly painful and problematic, while others were illuminating and transcendent. Suddenly the question of whether drugs can induce genuine religious and mystical experiences morphed from dry academic debates to pitched political battles with mainstream naysayers largely winning. Consequently there is currently a tendency to deny religious significance to any drug experience.

And yet the question—one of the most important of all concerning these curious chemicals—still remains: Can psychedelics induce genuine mystical experiences? Stanislav Grof, the world's most experienced psychedelic researcher, concluded that "after 30 years of discussion, the question of whether LSD and other psychedelics can induce genuine spiritual experiences is still open" (2001, 270).

At the present time both research and theory suggest an answer to this question. That answer is a very qualified "yes." Yes, psychedelics can induce genuine mystical experiences, but only *some* times, in *some* people, under *some* circumstances. To evaluate this conclusion, let's examine the arguments used against it, recent research, and a theory that makes sense of the research.

ARGUMENTS AGAINST THE VALIDITY OF DRUG-INDUCED RELIGIOUS EXPERIENCES

Five major arguments have been advanced against the idea that drug experiences can be truly religious or mystical.

1. Some drug experiences are clearly anything but mystical and beneficial.
2. The experiences induced by drugs may actually be different from those of genuine mystics.
3. A theological argument claims that mystical rapture is a gift of God, which can never be brought under mere human control.
4. The fourth argument is that drug-induced experiences are too quick and easy and could therefore hardly be identical to those hard won by years of contemplative discipline.

5. Finally, the aftereffects of drug-induced experiences may be different, less beneficial, and less long lasting than those of contemplatives.

There are possible answers to each of these concerns. Let's consider them in sequence.

1. There is no doubt whatsoever that some, in fact most, drug experiences are anything but mystical. According to Huston Smith:

> There are, of course, innumerable drug experiences that have no religious features; they can be sensual as readily as spiritual, trivial as readily as transforming, capricious as readily as sacramental. If there is one point about which every student agrees, it is that there is no such thing as the drug experience per se. . . . This of course proves that not all drug experiences are religious; it does not prove that no drug experiences are religious. (1964, 520)

2. Are drug and natural mystical states experientially the same? Smith concludes that "descriptively drug experiences cannot be distinguished from their natural religious counterparts" (523). In philosophical terms, drug and natural mystical experiences can be phenomenologically (experientially) indistinguishable. The most dramatic experiment affirming this was the "Harvard Good Friday study," also known as "the miracle of Marsh Chapel." In this study, divinity students and professors were placed in a spiritually supportive setting—Boston University's Marsh Chapel during a Good Friday service—and given either the psychedelic psilocybin or a placebo. Several psilocybin subjects reported "mystical experiences," which researchers could not distinguish from those of mystics throughout the centuries.

   Perhaps the people best equipped to decide whether drug and contemplatively induced mystical experiences might be the same are those who have had both. Such people are obviously few and far between. However, several spiritual teachers and scholars have concluded from their personal experience that they can be identical.

3. The third argument—that mystical rapture is a gift from God that could never be brought under human control—will seem plausible only to people who hold very specific theological beliefs. It would hardly be regarded as valid by religions such as Buddhism, for example, that do not believe in an all-powerful creator God. Nor, presumably, would it appeal to those theists who believe more in the power of good works than of grace.

4. The complaint that drug experiences are too easy to be genuine is readily understandable. After all, it hardly seems fair that a contemplative should labor for decades for a sip of what the psychedelic user may effortlessly swim in for hours. However, unfair or not, if the states are experientially identical, then the fact that they are due to different causes may be irrelevant. Technically this is called "the principle of causal indifference." Simply stated, this means that subjectively identical experiences can be produced by multiple causes.

5. The final argument against the equivalence of drug and natural mystical states is that they can have different long-term effects. Specifically, drug experiences may sometimes result in less profound, less enduring, or less beneficial transformations of personality and behavior. Once again Huston Smith put the case eloquently: "Drugs appear to induce religious experiences: it is less evident that they can produce religious lives" (1964, 528–29).

A THEORETICAL FRAMEWORK

So it seems that drug and natural mystical experiences can be subjectively similar, or even identical, yet still sometimes differ in their aftereffects. Yet the debate still continues over whether psychedelically induced mystical experiences are "really genuine."

One reason the debate continues unabated is that there has been no theory of mystical states that could resolve it. What is needed is a theory accounting for the induction of similar or identical states by such means as LSD and meditation, followed by possible different aftereffects.

Charles Tart's 2001 systems model of consciousness is helpful here. Tart suggests that any one state of consciousness is the result of the function and interaction of many psychological and neural processes, such as perception, attention, emotions, and identity. If any one process is changed sufficiently, it may shift the entire mind-brain system and state of consciousness. For example, a yogi might focus unwaveringly on the breath, a Christian contemplative might cultivate the love of God, or a Sufi might recite the name of Allah (*dhikr*). Yet despite their different practices, all might eventually be rewarded with mystical experiences, though not necessarily identical ones.

Whether different traditions can induce identical mystical experiences and in what ways their experiences may differ is a complex debate. For arguments that the experiences of different traditions are necessarily different see Stephen Katz (ed.), *Mysticism and Religious Traditions* (1983). For arguments that they can overlap see Robert Forman (ed.), *The Problem of Pure Consciousness* (1997); Huston Smith, *Forgotten Truth* (1997); Roger Walsh and Frances Vaughan (eds.), *Paths Beyond Ego* (1993); and Ken Wilber, *Integral Psychology* (2000). Clearly there are multiple kinds of religiously induced mystical experiences, just as there are multiple kinds of psychedelic experiences. Fortunately we don't need to go into these complexities to investigate whether some psychedelic experiences may overlap some mystical experiences.

A specific altered state can be reached in several ways by altering different processes. For example, states of calm may be reached by reducing muscle tension, visualizing restful scenery, repeating a pacifying thought, focusing attention on the breath, or taking a tranquilizer. In each case the brain-mind process used is different, but the resulting state is similar, a convergence that systems theorists call "equifinality."

A similar phenomenon may occur with mystical states. Different techniques might affect different brain-mind processes yet still result in a similar ASC. A Christian contemplative might finally taste the bliss of mystical unity after years of reciting the Jesus prayer; a karma yogi after decades of selfless service, and a Buddhist after long practice of insight meditation. Yet a psychedelic might modify chemical and neural processes so powerfully as to temporarily induce a similar state.

So Tart's theory of consciousness may provide an explanation for the finding that "chemical mysticism" and natural mysticism can be experientially identical. But what of the claim for differing long-term effects? This claim is also compatible with the theory. But first we need to consider whether the claim that the long-term effects of chemical mysticism are less beneficial and enduring is actually true.

LONG-TERM EFFECTS AND STABILIZATION

Contrary to common arguments, psychedelic mysticism *can* sometimes have enduring benefits. For example, in 2000 Huston Smith described just such an impact on himself, as did the psychologist Frances Vaughan in 1983, while Sherana Harriette Frances portrayed hers in a series of exquisite drawings in 2001. Research studies also suggest possible long-term benefits. Significant numbers of Buddhist retreatants were drawn to spiritual practice following psychedelics (Tart 1991). Likewise, for the most famous of all studies—the Harvard Good Friday study in which researchers could not distinguish the experimental subjects' psilocybin-induced mystical experiences from classical natural experiences. When the subjects were interviewed more than twenty years later, most of them reported that their psilocybin experience had contributed to their spiritual lives, and some still regarded the experience as one of the most important of their lives.

But even if we were to assume that the drugs have relatively little long-term benefit, is this so surprising? Or is it so different from other powerful experiences? After all, the stabilization of transient experiences and insights into enduring change is one of the great challenges facing all transformative disciplines. Psychoanalysts say "insight is not enough," while clinical psychologists speak of breakthroughs and regressions and of the "problem of generalization," that is, the problem of getting insights on the couch to generalize to daily life. Likewise, learning theorists describe "spontaneous recovery," whereby newly learned behavior fades and old patterns revive. It is true that powerful experiences can *sometimes* induce dramatic, enduring "quantum change." Yet, most people suffer from "false hope syndrome" and underestimate just how hard it is to change ingrained habits.

The same is true of religious disciplines. Profound experiences can *sometimes* effect enduring changes, but all too often these fade unless stabilized by further practice, as Philip Kapleau made clear in 1965 for *The Three Pillars of Zen*.

> Even the Buddha continued to sit. Without *joriki,* the particular power developed through *zazen* [seated meditation], the vision of oneness attained in enlightenment in time becomes clouded and eventually fades into a pleasant memory instead of remaining an omnipresent reality shaping our daily life. To be able to live in accordance with what the mind's eye has revealed through *satori* requires, like the purification of character and the development of personality, a ripening period of *zazen*. (Quoted in Smith 2000, 31)

A single spiritual experience is certainly no guarantee of a spiritual life or an ethical lifestyle. However, long-term practice and multiple experiences can have a cumulative impact. Enduring change usually requires enduring practice. So the limited long-term effects of psychedelic mystical experiences are far from unique. Rather, they reflect one of the central problems of psychological and spiritual growth: the "problem of stabilization."

But let's assume the critics' position. Let's assume for the moment that chemical mysticism is less transformative than contemplative mysticism, as well it might be. Why might this be so? Psychological, social, and spiritual factors may all be involved. Psychedelic users may have dramatic experiences, perhaps the most dramatic of their entire lives. However, a single experience, no matter how powerful, may be insufficient to permanently overcome mental and neural habits conditioned for decades to mundane modes of functioning.

A shaman or contemplative, on the other hand, may spend decades deliberately working to retrain habits along more spiritual lines. Thus, when the breakthrough finally occurs, it visits a mind already prepared for it. The contemplative probably has a belief system to make sense of the experience, a tradition that values it, a discipline to cultivate it, a social group to support it, and an ethic to guide it. As Louis Pasteur said, "Chance favors the prepared mind." The contemplative's mind may be prepared, but there is no guarantee that a drug user's is.

Therefore, different long-term effects of chemical and contemplative experiences could occur, even if the original experiences are identical. Consequently, none of the five common arguments against psychedelic experiences being genuinely mystical seem to hold.

CONCLUSION

In summary, it seems that psychedelics can induce genuine mystical experiences in some people on some occasions. However, they may be more likely to do so, and more likely to yield enduring benefits, when used as part of a long-term spiritual practice that prepares the mind beforehand and stabilizes insights afterward. This is exactly how traditional spiritual practitioners such as shamans use psychedelics, and therefore it is not surprising that many shamans value them as important aids to spiritual life and healing work.

6

Do Psychedelic-induced Mystical Experiences Boost the Immune System?

We know that when our lives are going well, when our relationships are running smoothly, and when we are achieving in our jobs, these life contexts make us happy and strengthen our immune systems. These emotionally positive events in people's daily lives are weaker forms of similar experiences that occur during mystical states, leading to the hypothesis that psychedelic-induced mystical experiences boost the immune system. While confirmation or disconfirmation of the hypothesis needs to come from experimental research, combined observations from biology, medicine, religion, psychology, and psychotherapy point to a fascinating relationship among psychedelic plants and chemicals, the mystical states they are capable of inducing under the right psychological state and physical location, and the immune system.

A tantalizing anecdote along these lines comes via Melissa Healy, a reporter for the *Los Angeles Times*. Ms. Healy reported that to reduce her anxiety about death—not to cure her underlying leukemia—a retired plant nursery worker became a volunteer in Griffiths's 2006 and 2008 psilocybin studies. Healy wrote:

Every three months, she gets her white blood cells checked. With her form of leukemia, those accounts are expected to rise steadily as the disease progresses. But in June 2009, four months after her psilocybin session, they went down. Every three months since, they have retreated further, leading two of her three doctors to declare her in remission.

This should not be overinterpreted. As the words say, spontaneous remissions usually happen on their own, without a mystical experience, but with further investigation this anecdote may become an early lead. And even if full remission does not always occur, the immune system might still be strengthened to a lesser extent by a psychedelic mystical experience.

There are many unknowns here, as suggested by my own varied entheogenic experiences: powerfully overwhelming states of unitive consciousness probably occurred about one-tenth of the time, while brief, more diluted episodes of a feeling of sacredness occurred over half the time, and strongly positive emotions most of the time. Given the ten- to twelve-hour duration of LSD experiences, most sessions have a mixture of thoughts, feelings, perceptions, and so forth.

These mixed results prompt the first of several caveats about the hypothesis. First, this hypothesis does not apply to *all* psychedelic usage nor to *all* religious uses but only to those occasions when psychedelics bring about states characterized by profound mystical experiences, particularly a sense of oneness. Some religions use marijuana sacramentally, but this usage does not seem to produce states of unitive consciousness and thus falls short of the mystical state that is an essential element of this hypothesis.

Also, this idea does not apply to *psycholytic* psychotherapy, which uses small doses of LSD, often in multiple sessions, as a way to help bring otherwise blocked material to consciousness. Because the small doses, used as an adjunct to usual psychotherapeutic practices, do not produce a mystical experience, these instances are not covered by the hypothesis either. However, if the total psychotherapeutic process relieves the clients and patients of their problems, the release of tension, fear, anxiety, depression, and so on may show itself in an improved immune system as a result of a long-term better emotional life.

We can now test the relationships between mystical experiences and the immune system scientifically and clinically; such research will be aided by measurable factors, such as peak experiences and salivary IgA and insights provided by studies of other mindbody technologies.

THE PEAK-EXPERIENCE VARIABLE

High-dose, *psychedelic* psychotherapy, in contrast to low-dose psycholytic psychotherapy, uses single, heavy-dose sessions that have the intent of providing psychotherapeutic mystical experiences. Clinical researchers and therapists pretty consistently recognize the therapeutic effects of peak experiences.

In 1977, for example, while using psychedelics with cancer patients to help them reduce their fear of death, William Richards and colleagues found that the most significant variable in psychedelic psychotherapy is "the peak experience variable." In the 1960s and 1970s Richards was part of the original clinical research team at Maryland Psychiatric Research Center in Catonsville. Now he is one of the guides who stays with the volunteers during their sessions in the Johns Hopkins psilocybin studies, and he is a psychotherapist in private practice. The importance of the peak experience, or mystical experience, as the significant therapeutic event carried through to Charles Grob's 2011 study of reducing anxiety in dying patients.

The fact that high-dose therapy does not always produce a state of unitive consciousness could be useful in studying the hypothesis. Conceivably, if the predominant emotions raised by the therapy were negative and if the patients' stress were unresolved, "unsuccessful" high-dose sessions would provide a comparison to mystical-experience sessions: both would be high-dose but with opposite emotional tones. Frequently, high-dose psychedelic sessions are a mixture of extreme emotions, both positive and negative. How these would affect the immune system is anybody's guess. My guess is that the final emotional state will be most influential.

A HELPFUL INDICATOR: SALIVARY IMMUNOGLOBULIN A

Probably the easiest way to evaluate the immune system is by taking a saliva sample and measuring its immunoglobulin A (IgA). IgA is the major immunoglobulin in the fluids that bathe the mucosal surfaces of the body (e.g., tears, saliva, gastrointestinal, vaginal, nasal, and bronchial secretions) and the surfaces that are the paths of entry into the body for invading bacteria and viruses. IgA is only one of the immune system's defenses—there are other immune indicators that might lend themselves to study as well—but salivary IgA is especially easy to sample, because it has the advantage of being readily obtainable while causing a minimal disruption to an ongoing psychedelic session. Its use is especially appropriate during a situation when suggestibility is heightened and subjects may be easily frightened or stressed by blood-taking procedures. And saliva sampling would not be beyond the professional qualifications and personal preferences of many potential researchers into this area, including theologians, psychologists, and sociologists.

Besides the ease of taking a sample, another reason for using salivary measures, and specifically IgA, as indicators of the immune system's health is the large number of studies that form a theoretical background and empirical base for doing so. In their 1992 review *Saliva as a Diagnostic Fluid,* Glock, Heller, and Malamud list 2,298 citations from more than 7,500 that they initially retrieved. Of these, 174 consider immunoglobulins. From 1993 through September 1998, *Medline*—the premier bibliographic database of the National Library of Medicine, which identifies itself as "The World's Largest Medical Library"—lists 6,486 IgA citations, some salivary, some not. From 1998 to 2011 it lists 14,723 IgA studies. Of those, 11,046 were in humans. Thus salivary IgA studies are embedded in a widely recognized research base with established methods and professional practices.

From the perspective of the hypothesis that psychedelic-induced mystical experiences boost the immune system, a problem with these salivary IgA studies is that only a small fraction address wellness, positive health, or positive experiences: only 287 studies included mood and only 43 looked for positive mood. However, there are intriguing research leads that link stressful daily events with lower salivary IgA levels and positive events with higher levels. For example, in a series of studies by Stone et al. (1987, 1994, 1996), desirable and undesirable daily events were found to influence IgA up or down, respectively.

IMPACTS OF MINDBODY PSYCHOTECHNOLOGIES

Among the many mindbody psychotechnologies that can improve emotions, positive mood-enhancing chemicals get the short end of the research stick in IgA research. Imagery, relaxation training, music, laughter, group support, talking therapy, movies with positive emotions, meditation, and therapeutic touch all show improved immune strength, but they are within the usual range of positive emotions, not at the possible psychedelic extremes.

Imagery is one of the better studied mindbody techniques. In *Complementary and Alternative Medicine*, Lyn Freeman summarizes the imagery research. "These studies suggest that children are more immediately susceptible to imagery as a method for altering certain parameters of immune function, but adults can also be trained to modulate immune function when more practice is provided" (2009, 260–63). Harman's 1966 study and other indications of links between psychedelics and creative problem solving suggest that psychedelics and imagery could be a natural pair that would strengthen each other. The positive suggestion of healing imagery to clients by psychedelic session monitors might enhance the capability of both of these mindbody psychotechnologies to improve immune function.

Thanks to increasing acceptance of complementary alternative medicine, health care in general may provide a warmer atmosphere for mindbody approaches to health. In his 2011 article in *Archives of Internal Medicine,* David Alfandre reported, "More than a third of Americans use some form of complementary and alternative medicine (CAM) and that number continues to rise attributed mostly to increases in the use of mind-body therapies (MBT) like yoga, meditation and deep breathing exercises" (1,685). The lead researcher, Dr. Aditi Nerurkar, Integrative Medicine Fellow at Harvard Medical School and at Beth Israel Deaconess Medical Center, evaluated survey data from more than 23,393 U.S. households. Finding that medical practitioners are increasingly referring their patients for nonstandard treatments, he and his coauthors summarized, "There's good evidence to support using mind-body therapies clinically" (Nerurkar et al. 2011, 864).

But what about exceedingly positive emotions? With the ultimate, most intense positive mood occurring in mystical experiences, it seems likely that they will boost the immune system even more. But psychedelics should not be taken for that reason until there is solid evidence that they do. The whole issue of the possible immune effects of exceedingly positive experiences is not clear, because all scientific research done to date has been within the range of normal daily events. The immune effects of exceedingly strong positive affect have yet to be studied. Even when they are studied it will likely be in medical research clinics with their careful screening, extensive preparation, and controlled environment. So their findings may not generalize to unscreened people in random settings. To adapt common TV warnings: "This is done by trained professionals. Do not try this at home."

Even if psychedelic-induced mystical experiences strengthen immune functions, it may be only to a marginal degree. As Stone and his co-investigators found in a 1987 study of IgA, the role of positive emotions may be primarily to counteract negative emotions; the positive emotions may not actually add strength to the immune system beyond its normal capacity. When Valdimarsdottir and Bovbjerg looked at the increase in natural killer cell activity during positive moods, they found that the benefits seemed related to positive moods when overcoming negative moods, raising the possibility again "that positive mood may

moderate, or buffer, the effects of negative mood on immune function"
(1997, 319). That is, positive mood may or may not strengthen natural
killer cell activity beyond its normal range.

COMPARING MYSTICAL EXPERIENCE AND CASES OF SPONTANEOUS REMISSION

Such cautions and caveats notwithstanding, in seeking to answer the
question of whether the powerful positive affects and cognitions during mystical experiences strengthen the immune system a great deal,
we may be aided by investigating the similarities between the cluster of
effects that occur during spontaneous mystical experiences, psychedelic-
induced mystical experiences, and spontaneous remissions.

As mentioned in chapter 2, in philosophy, religious studies, and the
psychology of religion, "mystical experience" denotes a specific experience or a group of similar experiences. In the *Journal of Religion and
Health,* Pahnke and Richards listed nine subjective experiences: (1) a
feeling of oneness, that is, ego transcendence; (2) objectivity and reality—
noetic quality or sense of truth; (3) a transcendence of time and space;
(4) a feeling of sacredness; (5) deeply felt positive mood; (6) an awareness of paradoxicality—an awareness that is anomalous in the Western
scientific paradigm; (7) a feeling that the experience is ineffable; (8)
transiency; and (9) positive changes in attitude or behavior (1966). They
can be elaborated to include any of the following experiences: transcendence, self-transcendence, temporary ego loss, ego transcendence, unitive consciousness, oneness with the universe, cosmic consciousness,
no-self, divine grace, divine rapture, religious conversion experience,
peak experience, mystical unity, and others.

Thanks to Hood's construction of a mysticism scale in 1975 and
its subsequent modifications and also to the concurrent growth of
transpersonal psychology, there is a substantial amount of empirical
research on mystical experiences. Three summaries of the literature
show that mystical experiences tend to be associated with indicators
of positive mental health. Because most of these findings come from

correlational studies, it is not clear whether mystical experiences help produce these characteristics, intensify already existing traits, or occur because of a third factor such as someone's personality. Future experimental studies with psychedelics might help clear up this theoretical ambiguity. In any event, for us the critical question is whether the characteristics of mystical experiences correlate with improved functioning of the immune system.

Psychospiritual and Psychosocial Boosts for the Immune System

If psychedelic mystical experiences share characteristics with other events that enhance salivary IgA (sIgA), it is entirely reasonable to hypothesize that they provide the link. We need to keep in mind that most of the treatments tried so far as interventions to enhance sIgA are presumed to reduce stress. That is, they reduce negative emotions rather than increase positive emotions to boost the immune system. This is in keeping with contemporary medicine's orientation to curing illness rather than supporting health and wellness. Coping with negative mood may not be the same as increasing positive mood, especially increasing positive mood to the great extremes occurring during some kinds of mystical experiences. Nevertheless, the reduction of unpleasant emotions, depression, and other stressful daily events that weaken the immune system as measured by sIgA represent, in essence, an increase in positive mood.

In a killer-cell study done in 2008, Masahiro Matsunaga and twelve coauthors measured simultaneously recorded brain, endocrine, and immune activities when positive emotions were evoked as people watched films featuring their favorite persons. "These results suggest that while an individual experiences positive emotions, the central nervous, endocrine, and immune systems may be interrelated, and attraction for favorite persons may be associated with the activation of the innate immune function via the dopaminergic system" (408). On the other hand, working with an apparently healthy and nonstressed group of school-age children, Lambert and Lambert discovered that concentrations of salivary IgA were increased after a humorous presentation, raising the possibility that the presentation strengthened this immune component beyond its normal range (1995).

In "Psychosocial Factors and Secretory Immunoglobulin A," Doctors Valdimarsdottir and Stone selected and summarized about two dozen research studies on the relationships between sIgA and both stressful events and stress-reduction interventions. Although the authors cautioned that "methodological refinements are needed before more definitive conclusions can be made," they maintained that the studies indicated that various stress-reduction interventions are associated with increases in salivary IgA levels (1997). The question that concerns us is whether the interventions that increase salivary IgA exhibit—perhaps in a weakened form—characteristics that also appear in mystical experiences.

The stress-reduction techniques that have been tried include relaxation response, progressive relaxation, guided visualization, imaging powerful immune functions, back massage, music combined with a self-induced state of appreciation, self-hypnosis, suggestions, and humorous movies. These interventions are consistent with the decreased need for ego defensiveness that accompanies ego-transcendent states and feelings of belonging and unity as well as a deeply felt positive mood—all characteristics of mystical experiences. Further, on the basis of the assumption that human abilities vary in strength from one mindbody state to another, visualization, suggestion, hypnosis, and imaging are probably more powerful in some altered mindbody states, an important possibility considering that psychedelics alter mindbody states.

In short, although studies of the results of these interventions do not directly investigate the relationship between mystical states and improved immune function, as a whole they are in the expected direction, and these stress-reduction interventions look like mild examples of more powerful psychedelic interventions. The most common feature of both types of interventions is positive emotions.

Studies of social support offer another possible link to the characteristics of mystical experiences. For example, Jemmott and Magloire found that high levels of sIgA are associated with social support. For people who have had mystical experiences, the feelings of unity, belonging in the universe, being cared for, and "coming to one's ultimate home" provide feelings of extreme support, even cosmic support. Cosmic belonging such as feeling in the hands of God may substitute, and even more than substitute, for ordinary, interpersonal social support (1988).

Studies of social support, positive psychological mood, and desirable daily events show all three are correlated with increased sIgA. These studies also provide some general support for a link between positive experience and increased sIgA.

Mystical States and Spontaneous Remission

Let us ratchet up the importance of the possible significance of the psychedelic-unitive-immune hypothesis. If positive day-to-day experiences strengthen the immune system somewhat, might powerfully positive experiences—mystical states, states of unitive consciousness, ego-transcendent states—strengthen the immune system powerfully, even to the point of being associated with unusual cures? Some suggestive data prompts this question.

In their 1993 *Spontaneous Remission: An Annotated Bibliography,* O'Regan and Hirshberg presented a table of "Psychospiritual Correlates of Remission" (see page 98). Their list resembles both the characteristics of mystical experiences and of daily events, moods, and attitudes that are associated with increased levels of salivary IgA.

Many of the twenty-seven psychospiritual correlates shown in the table are characteristics of both mystical experiences and events that boost salivary IgA. Others, such as a sense of belonging, discarding ego centeredness, reorienting one's life, and altered states of consciousness are typical of mystical experiences but do not appear in sIgA research. The correlates that emphasize insights into one's personal life and social relationships parallel the results of decreased ego attachment that often follow ego transcendence, both psychedelic and nonpsychedelic. Another cluster of correlates is composed of experiences of altered-states phenomena—the very nature of mystical experience.

Common Correlates of Spontaneous Remission

(based on *Spontaneous Remission* by O'Regan and Hirshberg)

Group support

Hypnosis/suggestion

Meditation

Relaxation techniques

Mental imagery

Psychotherapy/psychoanalysis

Behavioral therapy

Group therapy

Miraculous spiritual phenomena

Prayer/spiritual belief

Religious/spiritual conversion

Autonomous behavior/increased autonomy

Faith/positive outcome expectancy

Fighting spirit

Denial

Lifestyle/attitude/behavioral (changes)

Social relationships/interpersonal relationship/family support

Positive emotions/acceptance of negative emotions

Environmental/social awareness/altruistic

Expression of needs/demands/self-nurturing

Sense of control/internal locus of control

Desire/will to live

Increased or altered sensory perception

Taking responsibility for the illness

Sense of purpose

Placebo effect

Diet/exercise

Taking such parallels into consideration, might it be reasonable to say that there is a persistent cluster of feelings, thoughts, moods, and behaviors that occur in mystical experiences, in daily events associated with increased sIgA levels, and in spontaneous remission? This is a great question for future researchers to investigate. At this point, an inclination toward a positive answer can be only conjecture. O'Regan and Hirshberg report disappointingly few findings that show a relationship between mystical states and unaccountable cures. (Given that both spontaneous remissions and mystical experiences occur at low rates in a population, this may not be so surprising.) Still, they provide some suggestive clinical observations.

They note that at the first conference on spontaneous regression held at Johns Hopkins in 1974, Dr. Renee Mastrovito of the neuropsychiatric service at Memorial Sloan Kettering Cancer Center alluded to historical references to cures following religious conversion or prayer. They also point to a study by Ikemi and others of five selected cases "who made a narrow escape from cancer" (1975). According to O'Regan and Hirshberg, the authors claim that the patients' spontaneous cures were supported and encouraged by their religious faith or favorable change of human environment (social relationship) and suggest that the background of Asian thought also might help them reach such a blessed state of mind. In three of the five cases "the unchanged or rather elevated immunological capacity which was usually lowered in cancer patients has been confirmed" (O'Regan and Hirshberg 1993).

A comment on another survey of eighteen cases of cancer regression by Weinstock aligned the typical feelings of hope, purpose, and meaning that follow mystical experiences with recovery. "All 18 definitely did not have anything for which to live before the favorable psychosocial change, and all found life very much worth living afterwards" (1983). The 2006 and 2008 Johns Hopkins psilocybin studies provide a lead on how to boost meaningfulness and other positive thoughts and emotions. O'Regan and Hirshberg also cite clinical reports by Meares of twelve cases of spontaneous regression of cancers associated with intensive meditation. In the discussion of one case, Meares wrote, "It may well be that the extreme reduction of anxiety in these patients triggers off the mechanism which becomes active in the rare spontaneous remissions. This would be consistent with the observation that spontaneous remissions are often associated with some kind of religious experience or profound psychological reaction" (1979, 540).

We can suppose that the religious conversion experiences, blessed states of mind, and marked favorable psychosocial change reported in the studies above probably indicate strongly felt positive moods and possibly peak or ego-transcendent mystical experiences. From a transpersonal perspective a consistent source of psychological anxiety and its resulting physical stress is overidentification with the ego. Might it be that ego transcendence or dis-identification during meditation and mystical experiences contribute to spontaneous remission?

This is not to say that all, or even most, spontaneous remissions occur via mystical experiences. In their 2004 study of eleven people who experienced spontaneous remissions of cancer, Schilder, de Veies, Goodkin, and Antoni found that changes that preceded remissions were "more day to day life, living in the here and now, with sometimes simple, yet for that person basic and meaningful acts and feelings" (Schilder 2011). Remissions based on mystical experiences may be a special class, not the general case.

SUMMARY—TAKING UP UNFINISHED WORK

What is the answer to the question with which we started this chapter? If positive day-to-day experiences strengthen the immune system somewhat, might powerfully positive experiences strengthen the immune system powerfully, even to the point of contributing to unusual cures and spontaneous remissions? "Maybe" or "I hope so" are not very satisfying answers, but considering the current state of knowledge, they are probably the most accurate ones.

In their summary of psychosocial factors affecting sIgA, Valdimarsdottir and Stone conclude that both negative and positive affect mediate between daily events and sIgA levels. This "indicates that researchers should not only focus on the role of negative affect but should also consider the contribution of positive affect" (1997, 470). This chapter's hypothesis adds, "Especially extremely powerful positive affect." More than thirty years ago in *Psychedelic Drugs Reconsidered,* the book-length review of the scientific and scholarly literature (more than 1,000 studies), Grinspoon and Bakalar summarized their position:

After more than ten years of almost total neglect, it is time to take up the work that was laid down unfinished in the sixties. We need to arrange a way for people to take psychedelic drugs responsibly under appropriate guidance within the law, and a way for those who want to administer them to volunteers for therapeutic and general research to do so. (1975, 293)

They wrote this after reviewing nearly the whole body of psychedelic research in anthropology, psychotherapy, religion, creativity, medicine, psychology, and related fields. Now, three decades later, work is beginning to progress again, and this chapter adds a question that gives a new reason to restart this research: Do entheogen-induced mystical experiences boost the immune system?

I would like to thank Johannes N. Schilder for his perceptive and insightful critique of this chapter.

The next chapter, "Psychedelic Psychotherapy Near the End of Life," looks at current research into the use of psychedelics to reduce fear of death in people with terminal illness and speculates about how and why this use seems likely. Unlike pain killers and drugs that cloud consciousness, the key is mystical experience. In this second guest chapter, psychiatrist Charles Grob and his coresearcher and coauthor Alicia Danforth describe their pilot study of using psilocybin as an adjunct to treatment for fear of death. What do psychedelics say about dying? Grob, Danforth, and their patients describe how the combination of psychotherapy and intense psilocybin experiences can ease this transition. Is this a clue to hospice treatments of the future?

7

Psychedelic Psychotherapy Near the End of Life

CHARLES S. GROB, M.D., AND ALICIA L. DANFORTH

Charles S. Grob, M.D., is professor of psychiatry and pediatrics at the UCLA School of Medicine and director of the Division of Child and Adolescent Psychiatry at Harbor-UCLA Medical Center. Alicia Danforth is finishing her Ph.D. in clinical psychology from the Institute of Transpersonal Psychology.

Death must become a more human experience. To preserve the dignity of death and prevent the living from abandoning or distancing themselves from the dying is one of the great dilemmas of modern medicine.

SIDNEY COHEN, M.D., 1965

For individuals approaching the end of life, severe and persistent spiritual and existential crises are common occurrences. Even though modern medicine has progressed considerably in developing effective treatments for advanced-stage disease, often extending survival time for months or even years, efforts designed to address the psychological distress of terminal illness have often been limited (Cassel 1982). Indeed, conventional state-of-the-art psychiatric treatment for advanced-stage cancer clients, particularly the commonly administered selective serotonin re-uptake inhibitors (SSRIs), a class of antidepressants, have failed to demonstrate positive effects on anxiety, mood, and quality of life in carefully designed research investigations (Stockler et al. 2007). Recently, however, increasing interest has been directed toward understanding and treating the spiritual and existential crises that individuals near the end of life frequently encounter (Rousseau 2000; Breitbart et al. 2004; McCoubrie and Davies 2006).

Surveys have found that up to 70 percent of individuals with advanced-stage cancer experience heightened and often clinically significant anxiety. Depression and despair in cancer clients is not uncommon and leads to poorer survival rates, suicidal preoccupation and behavior, desire for hastened death, and requests for physician-assisted suicide. Existential anxiety, while a universal phenomena, develops greater intensity and urgency at the end of life, along with heightened perception of vulnerability and inevitable death. The profound spiritual suffering often experienced as individuals approach the end of life shares many features of severe depression, including hopelessness, worthlessness, meaninglessness, social isolation, anger, guilt, and remorse. Addressing such conditions of spiritual and existential distress encourages active life review, along with a realistic appreciation of current realities and assists in recognizing purpose, value, meaning, forgiveness, and reconciliation.

The great challenge for individuals nearing the end of their lives is often one of sustaining a sense of meaning and purpose. As the physical body declines and approaches death, individuals are often overwhelmed with pain and suffering, psychological as well as physical, and they begin to lose the thread of meaning and coherence that had previously defined their lives. By addressing spiritual needs, however, another dimension is added that allows for a focus on the need for love and good relationships with self and others, along with the need for forgiveness, hope, joy, peace, dignity, and trust. Exploring spiritual concerns also allows individuals the potential to rise above present circumstances and to engage positively with other people, surroundings, and powers outside of the self, irrespective of the presence or absence of religious belief systems.

Transcendent experience, a vital component of spirituality, has the potential to take on greater subjective importance as a person nears the end of life. Encounters with transpersonal states of consciousness have generally been considered to be among the most powerful means by which a state of wholeness and personal integrity may be restored after serious psychological injury and end-of-life despair are alleviated.

PSYCHEDELIC PSYCHOTHERAPY

Psychedelic psychotherapy is a treatment approach that has been demonstrated to reliably facilitate enhanced states of spiritual transcendence and well-being when conducted under optimal conditions. The passage of time has allowed for a relaxing of restrictions imposed on research as a result of the cultural turmoil of the 1960s and has provided new opportunities to reexamine the range of safety and efficacy of this long-neglected treatment model.

The pioneers of psychedelic research several decades ago, along with more recent investigators, have made the practical determination that, when conducting hallucinogen-facilitated psychotherapy with advanced-stage cancer clients, it is important to adhere to certain structures that will increase the likelihood of positive outcome. To begin with, clients must be informed that the treatment will not cure their physical illness but may help them develop the emotional strength to cope with what lies ahead. A period of preparatory work is necessary to establish rapport and trust between the client and therapeutic team and to conduct a thorough life review, including an examination of past and current relationships. Communication issues are addressed, as are attitudes and fears of death and dying and concerns about the future (Pahnke 1969).

The treatment session is conducted in a pleasant and private setting, decorated with items such as tapestries, art, flowers, or objects that have meaning for the client. During the long psychedelic experience (four to six hours with psilocybin and eight to twelve hours with LSD), the client is encouraged to lie down, wearing an eyeshade while listening to preselected music through earphones (the experience of listening to music helps the client to let go of usual ego controls and experience a heightened degree of emotional awareness). Immediately after the session, family and friends may visit, as the post-session "afterglow" state often opens the opportunity for gratifying emotional interchanges. The final element of the treatment process is the integration of the experience, preferably with ongoing support from the research team, which occurs in the days, weeks, and months that follow.

Historical Research Background

Among the most promising areas of study coming out of the "Golden Age" of psychedelic research from the late 1950s to the early 1970s were a series of reports describing the work of investigators exploring the use of a psychedelic treatment model with clients who had been diagnosed with terminal cancer. Although he was not a medical researcher, the English literary figure Aldous Huxley was the first Western intellectual to identify the potential application of psychedelic compounds at the end of life. During the final ten years of his life, Huxley developed a fascination with the range of effects of the newly discovered psychedelics, and particularly in their potential to alleviate psychospiritual suffering. In his final work of fiction, *Island,* Huxley described the use of *moksha* (Sanskrit for "enlightenment") *medicine* to facilitate the passage of the terminally ill from life into death (Huxley 1962). True to his beliefs, Huxley arranged for his personal physician to inject him with 100 micrograms of LSD hours before he died.

Huxley was a close friend of Sidney Cohen, a prominent internist at the UCLA School of Medicine who developed the first program designed to examine the use of psychedelics to ameliorate the high levels of emotional distress often observed in patients dying of advanced medical illness. Unfortunately, the details of his findings were never reported. However, Cohen published the rationale for conducting this treatment in *Harper's Magazine* in 1965 in an article titled "LSD and the Anguish of Dying." Cohen fervently called for the development of a more effective intervention for individuals approaching the final stages of life, which he believed would one day alter the experience of dying (Cohen 1965).

The first clinician to make a rigorous effort to collect data on the effects of psychedelics in patients with serious medical illness was Eric Kast, an internist and pain specialist at Chicago Medical School. In a series of experiments during the early 1960s, Kast and his colleagues compared the efficacy of a modest dose of LSD, 100 micrograms, with standard narcotic medications used to treat pain, Demerol and Dilaudid. They found that the psychedelic's analgesic effects were superior to that obtained by the opiate derivatives. To their surprise they also observed that in the days and weeks after receiving LSD some of their patients displayed "a striking disregard for the gravity of their personal situations. They frequently talked about their impending death with an emotional attitude that would be considered atypical in our culture; yet it was quite obvious that this new perspective was beneficial in view of the situation they were facing." Studying more than two hundred patients with terminal malignant disease, Kast found consistent and sustained improvements in physical pain, mood, and sleep. He also described the occurrence of "happy oceanic feelings," lasting up to twelve days following psychedelic administration. Improvements in morale and self-respect were evident, as were particular changes in philosophical and religious attitudes that appeared to noticeably lessen the fear of death (Kast 1966).

Stanislav Grof, a Czech psychiatrist with vast research experience in Europe, developed the most substantive program examining the application of a psychedelic treatment model with terminally ill clients. Grof had relocated in the late 1960s to the Maryland Psychiatric Research Center at Spring Grove State Hospital. Collaborating with Harvard-trained psychiatrist and theologian Walter Pahnke, he developed a rigorous approach to studying the range of psychospiritual effects in volunteer subjects with advanced-stage cancer. In their articles published in the professional literature, and later in Grof's book *The Human Encounter with Death* (cowritten with Joan Halifax) and *The Ultimate*

Journey, substantive evidence was presented demonstrating the efficacy and safety of the psychedelic treatment model when administered under optimal conditions. Findings included improved mood, reduced anxiety and reduced pain, and decreased need for narcotic medications. Investigators also identified that the best treatment outcomes occurred in subjects who, during the course of their psychedelic treatment, experienced a mystical or transpersonal (beyond ego) state of consciousness (Grof et al. 1973; Grof and Halifax 1977; Grof 2006).

Unfortunately, by the early 1970s political pressures forced the effective termination of all psychedelic research programs, including the groundbreaking work with advanced-cancer patients that Grof and his colleagues were conducting at Spring Grove. For years there was virtually no further discussion of the potential of the psychedelic treatment model to ameliorate the psychospiritual suffering of individuals close to death, although there was a gradual acceptance by society that greater attentiveness and sensitivity needed to be employed when caring for the terminally ill. Indeed, the advent of the hospice movement and the field of palliative medicine may in part have occurred owing to the work of these early psychedelic researchers. Nevertheless, three decades would elapse before sanctioned studies designed to evaluate the safety and efficacy of a psychedelic treatment model with clients with advanced-cancer anxiety would resume.

Current Research

Beginning in the early 1990s a few Phase I safety research investigations of hallucinogens were permitted in the United States, followed a decade later by several pilot clinical treatment trials. Recently, psilocybin in particular has been explored in an adjunctive therapeutic model with promising preliminary reports. Questions have been raised, however, concerning the choice of psilocybin in these studies over other classical or novel hallucinogens. One important advantage psilocybin has over the better-known LSD is that it carries less social stigma and consequently has a far less sensationalized reputation.

The more recently prominent drug MDMA, popularly known as

Ecstasy, also has been suggested as a possible treatment for cancer anxiety. However, the clear advantage of psilocybin over MDMA is its far safer range of cardiovascular effects. Although MDMA has therapeutic potential with people suffering from post-traumatic stress disorder, these are usually individuals in good physical health. On the other hand, clients with advanced cancer often have multiple organ system failures and are consequently more sensitive to the amphetamine-like effects of MDMA. Furthermore, psilocybin's greater capacity to catalyze transcendent and mystical states of consciousness would, according to the early investigators, lead to a more therapeutic outcome.

THE HARBOR-UCLA MEDICAL CENTER STUDY

From 2004 to 2008 a pilot research investigation conducted at Harbor-UCLA Medical Center explored the safety and feasibility of using psilocybin in research for participants with advanced cancer and associated anxiety. Of the twelve participants, eleven were female. The age range spanned from thirty-six to fifty-eight. Some participants had never taken a psychedelic drug, and others had varying levels of experience with them over many years. A double-blind, placebo-controlled investigative design was employed, with each subject receiving one psilocybin facilitated treatment experience and one with placebo. Safety was demonstrated when no subjects sustained physical or psychological injury from their psilocybin psychotherapy treatment (Grof et al. 1973; Grof and Halifax 1977; Grof 2006).

Participants had been living with a cancer diagnosis for an average of six years and four months by the time they volunteered for the study. Some of them were aware that cancer was likely to end their lives within one year, and some were still in the process of accepting that death was imminent. During enrollment screening the researchers listened carefully for indications that a potential participant was seeking a "miracle cure" for the cancer. They were all counseled in advance that the purpose of the study was not to treat or cure cancer but to assist them with anxiety and difficult emotions.

Results

A greater challenge was demonstrating efficacy of the treatment, which used only a moderate dose (0.2 mg/kg) of psilocybin. Quantitative psychological evaluations revealed some indications of therapeutic outcome. In particular, a significant reduction in one measure of anxiety was reported one month following treatment and was maintained for several additional months. Although a persistent change in another measure of anxiety was not reported, the assessment might reflect a sustained alteration in how subjects viewed their vulnerability to stress and anxiety over time. Subjects' mood also was noted to improve for a two-week period following treatment with psilocybin, with some indication of continued improvement up to the three months after treatment. While the study did not definitively establish therapeutic efficacy, results from this study were positive and supportive of still further investigation. With a larger cohort of subjects and use of a more robust dose of psilocybin, it seems likely that statistically significant results would be obtained on these measures.

Formal qualitative data gathering and content analysis methods were not included as part of this small study. However, notes from pre-session interviews, treatment session progress notes, and other written study records provide insight into the common subjective themes that emerged from participant experiences. Intentions for treatment were as variable as the life situations of the participants. All participants were encouraged during pre-session counseling to identify the main existential themes that were challenging for them, and often they chose intentions that were tangential to the direct fear and acknowledgment of the reality of dying earlier than anticipated. For example, several participants wanted to focus on the quality of their relationships with significant others or family members. Participants were encouraged to look inward and ask, "In spite of the likelihood that cancer was going to end life, what else remained to be healed and what meaning in life could be found until the moment when death occurred?"

Patient Reports

Several participants shared their personal experiences in writing on different qualities of healing they achieved as a result of participating in the study, during which they received psychedelic psychotherapy with psilocybin. Several of the themes that emerged are presented below in a progression from a focus on concerns of the body, then the mind, and finally to those of the spirit.

Body

Some of the participants reflected on body-based changes and new awarenesses that were achieved through undergoing psilocybin-assisted psychotherapy. In the following example a fifty-three-year-old female participant describes what she experienced during a rest room break while she was under the influence of psilocybin.

> I saw myself in the mirror while washing my hands and started to cry, grieving the effects of two rounds of chemotherapy: the loss of my long curly hair and my youthful looks. I talked about it a little with [the researchers]. After a while I felt acceptance. With loss of youth comes wisdom, greater ability to help others.

Because this and subsequent quotations come from private clinical records, their authors remain anonymous.

In another example from the same participant, psilocybin combined with music provided a reminder that, even in an ailing body, life still provided sources of enjoyment.

> I felt the music coursing through my body from my feet up to my head in ripples of energy. I danced lying down. I could feel it in every muscle. It was extremely enjoyable. I realized I need to make more music. My hands really want to play the flute again; I couldn't hold them still during one song, perhaps it had a flute in it.

Another participant in her middle fifties described a psilocybin-induced vision that supported her in the acceptance of the inevitability of departing her body.

> I scan my body as if from slightly above, checking to see how it is working. I see it is not. It is what I have been feeling, a shell. I pull back, higher, higher for a better view. My body is on a table and I am looking down from several feet. The right side of my body is nearly immobile. I see that it is heavy, starving, and inflexible. And then I see what, for some reason, doesn't surprise me: my body is done, I've outgrown it? Or it no longer can serve me as before? I like the feeling of leaving my body. I feel free. It weighs me down.

Issues of the body were especially relevant for this subject because she had been living on a liquid diet in a state of near starvation due to damage after treatment for head and neck cancer. However, she experienced an unexpected reprieve from her lack of ability to swallow solid food following psilocybin.

> For a short, amazing time two weeks after that journey, I was sitting at the kitchen table with my fiancé. He'd baked yams and fish. I picked up a fork and put a bit of yam in my mouth and waited to see if my throat would reject it, as usual, sending me running to the sink. This time, I swallowed the yam. Then some fish. My throat was a blossom opening. Every day I would sit with a small meal, a scrambled egg, some cheese, something soft. It had been so long since I'd eaten anything solid and I knew it was a gift. Soon enough, my throat began to atrophy again.

No medical conclusions can be drawn from anecdotes such as this one. However, this account raises interesting questions about the mind-body connection and the mechanisms by which psilocybin promotes different types of healing.

Mind

Some participants wrote about more inward-focused, cognitive-based shifts in thinking and attitudes that occurred as a result of psilocybin-assisted psychotherapy. They indicated that the range of subjective effects they encountered were often profound and valuable. Common themes included examining how their illness had impacted their lives, relationships with family and close friends, and sense of ontological security. Several subjects reported powerful empathic concentration on close friends and family members, whereas others examined how they wished to address their limited life expectancy optimally. The following account from a fifty-four-year-old female participant provides a sense of the type of new conscious awareness that psilocybin can catalyze.

> The experience taking the psilocybin for this study was new to me. I shunned mind-altering drugs in the past, though I grew up in the sixties. . . . I had an extremely deep, rich experience. The first feeling I had was happiness and I smiled, a lot, feeling that I "knew" life was to be taken that way. . . . I do know that my experience in this altered state lasted quite awhile and when I was made aware that it was ending, I was disappointed. I was comfortable, not afraid, and in touch with something that made me happy. I cannot say directly what long-lasting effect the one study had on me, because I value science and don't think I can make assumptions on one experience. I would very much like to repeat the study and compare experiences. . . . I remember thinking that life was funny and I could see the cosmic joke.

The female participant who contemplated body changes and the end of youth in the rest room mirror also described other mental shifts when she wrote, "I received reassurance that my doctors will control my pain with medication when the time comes. I will be able to handle it." And, "All of my questions have been answered. Who could ask for more than that?" In a letter to the lead investigator, the thirty-six-year-old male participant reflected on the benefit he received from new insights through psilocybin-assisted psychotherapy.

I just wanted to drop you a quick missive and thank you for the work that has been done with my psyche. I thoroughly enjoyed my experience and have retold the sequence of events probably thirty times so far. For a five hour investment, I'd feel hard pressed to walk away with more deep experiential learning. The work that [the researchers] are doing might not be right for everyone, but for the ones that can handle and learn from it, it is a godsend.

Several participants' primary focus for sessions, whether intended in advance of treatment or not, was on interpersonal concerns such as forgiveness, the pain of being the source of a partner's grief, fears about losing physical intimacy, and the strains on relationships of living with daily anxiety. The account below is from a fifty-three-year-old participant who reflected on a psilocybin-induced vision that helped her prepare to say good-bye to loved ones.

I am sitting in a circle with several Native Americans, a council it seems. They are telling me things. I find it interesting and soothing that this is all communicated through thought, no words spoken. We are surrounded by many animals. And then I am with my son and daughter, and I'm being told that there is but a short time when parent and child have the same strength and energy to do everything together, side by side. I am shown insights into my children that make huge sense to me. I begin scrolling faces of people I want to have better knowledge of—and I understand it is all there, everything I want to know, incredible insights into my loved ones and messages to pass along. And as I write these down in my notebook, my heart breaks open: I am writing farewell notes.

Spirit

In some cases participants reported nonordinary states of consciousness with the qualities of classic, numinous spiritual experiences. In fact, recent clinical research has shown psilocybin can be a reliable catalyst for mystical experiences. Pioneer investigators treating terminal cancer patients with hallucinogens in the 1960s and early 1970s identified that a key therapeutic outcome variable was the occurrence of a profound psychospiritual experience during the course of the hallucinogen treatment session (Grof et al. 1973; Grof and Halifax 1977). Accessing such transcendent states of consciousness is usually associated with higher dosages of hallucinogens, beyond the 0.2 mg/kg dose of psilocybin approved for the Harbor-UCLA study. Nevertheless, some participants sustained transpersonal states of consciousness.

> My first perception of the psilocybin's effects was a feeling of being supported by many hands. I did not know whose hands they were: perhaps [the Hindu deity] Avalokiteshvara, the plant spirits, or some universal spirit. I felt the sensation physically, as though the bed were not a bed but a circle of hands, supporting me. I felt with certainty that I had always and would always be held in that way.
>
> I felt the presence of spiritual guide(s) very strongly for several hours. . . . All seem to be giving me Buddhist teachings, probably due to my preconceived ideas about spirituality (but who knows?). They couldn't heal my cancer. They informed me that it's my karma to have cancer. This is part of my spiritual path—look how much it has taught me already. It's going to kill me eventually, I don't have control over that, but I can slow it down some.

In the months following treatment, participants often reflected on their altered state of consciousness experience and conveyed that they continued to derive benefit from the insights and new perspectives encountered while under the influence of psilocybin. This account from a fifty-three-year-old female was written eleven months after the psilocybin treatment.

> [While experiencing the effects of psilocybin,] I ask what has been my point of being here, on earth. There is no one point. I am and was and always will be. I feel elucidated! I understand that it never

really mattered what I did in terms of career, etc., just that I was living life to the fullest and that whatever I did reflected who I was. Though this is a foundation of nearly every spiritual belief system, hearing it again now, in this way, is so confirming, and a burden lifted. I wish I'd had the faith to believe this before. In the back of my mind all these years, I couldn't shake the idea that I thought I had to accomplish some thing in order to be fulfilled or to fulfill God's plan. No such thing. I am, was, always have been enough.

My journey was extraordinary. Though I have no doubt these altered states can be reached without drug-enhancement, this research offer from [the principal investigator] came at the perfect time for me. Meditation and concentration had become all but elusive since I'd been ill. Shifting attention away from the pain in my head and neck took every bit of my focus. But with the help of the mushroom, I was able to leap past the physical pain for a brief time and experienced a knowing that fills me daily with peace. I know I'm not going into a Void—there is God and life continuing.

Instead of gentle resignation to the inevitability of death, most participants experienced some degree of active reengagement with living in the time they had remaining. The forms this activation took were as various as the individuals. One mother called an adult child to return home from overseas. Another decided to stop taking prescription antidepressant medication, attributing the sustained improvement in mood to her psilocybin session. One couple credited psilocybin-assisted psychotherapy with possibly saving their marriage, which was strained under the pressures cancer brought to their daily lives. Canceled travels plans were put back on the calendar and enjoyed. One participant, who was living in an unsatisfactory situation with a former partner, found a new romance in the months before dying after a psilocybin-inspired revelation inspired a vision of an ideal partner.

CONCLUSION

After a hiatus of several decades there are encouraging signs that hallucinogen research is beginning to move forward again. Following the Harbor-UCLA psilocybin study, similar investigations have been initiated at Johns Hopkins and NYU. The promising findings of a previous generation of researchers now need to be replicated using contemporary state-of-the-art research methodologies. Early work with advanced-stage cancer clients in particular demonstrated the promise of effective intervention for psychospiritual crises often observed at the end of life. A critical element that is necessary to support such a program of research, which was not available to our predecessors but is to an increasing degree today, is a stable political and professional environment.

As there is renewed interest in clinical research with hallucinogens, great sensitivity must be utilized in selecting the psychotherapists who will do the actual work. It is imperative that, in addition to the requisite psychological acumen, therapists also possess sufficient emotional maturity, psychological stability, and ethical integrity to be able to conduct their work effectively and safely. Clients under the influence of hallucinogens are exquisitely sensitive to environmental stimuli, including the individual and collective input of the therapy team. Consequently, as both past and recent history attest, attentiveness to *set* (mental and emotional preparedness) and *setting* (ambiance, safety, support) remain paramount when conducting clinical investigations with hallucinogens (Fisher 1970). Given the universality of the essential existential dilemma, and the potential for the optimally conducted hallucinogen treatment model to improve the quality of the end of life period, there is clearly a need to develop further research that will demonstrate the utility of this field of hallucinogen medicine.

LINKS TO RELATED VIDEOS AND WEBSITES

On page 117 we've provided a list of websites that we find to be the most informative regarding clinical research and psychedelics.

"The Use of Hallucinogens in Psychiatry and Medicine"
www.maps.org/videos/source/video13.html
The authors' presentation on the Harbor-UCLA psilocybin cancer anxiety study, April 2010, at the MAPS Psychedelic Science in the Twenty-first Century conference, San Jose, California.

Heffter Research Institute, "Harbor—UCLA Psilocybin & Cancer"
www.heffter.org/research-hucla.htm
See an interview with Pam Sakuda, a psilocybin study participant, at the Department of Psychiatry, Harbor-UCLA Medical Center, Torrance, California.

Documentary Jukebox, "Annie's Psilocybin Therapy"
www.doc-jukebox.com/film/medical-research-psychedelics/annies-psilocybin-therapy
This video provides an excerpt from "THE MEDICINE: Science & Psychedelics—'Annie's Psilocybin Therapy,'" documenting Annie Levy's experience in Charles Grob's UCLA psilocybin treatment for terminally ill cancer patients research study.

ClinicalTrials.gov, "Psilocybin Cancer Anxiety Study"
http://clinicaltrials.gov/ct2/show/NCT00957359
This link provides information about the New York University psilocybin cancer anxiety study, including participant eligibility criteria and contact information.

Johns Hopkins Medicine, "Psilocybin Cancer Project"
www.cancer-insight.org
This link provides information about the Johns Hopkins psilocybin cancer anxiety study.

PART 2

High-Yield Ideas

Multistate Theory and the Fruitful Mind

Psychedelics are more than a door to perception, more than a doorway to the numinous, more than an adjunct to psychotherapy, and more than a portal to the religion of direct experience. They are also entrances to rich idea mines.

In part 1 we focused on one state, the mystical state (although, to be more exact, some people regard mystical experiences as a collection of similar states, ones that overlap a great deal). Part 1 illustrates how experiencing that state commonly affects our values, spiritual development, fear of death, and possibly even our immune systems. Because mystical states and psychedelic effects are too powerful to ignore, they are one undeniable example of how different states and ways of producing them influence our minds and who we are.

However, when we look back at chapters 1 through 7, a bigger question begs to be asked: "Are psychedelics and mystical experiences unique, or are they windows to something more, something bigger? Are they one example of a larger class of things?" In part 2 we see that these states and the psychedelic way of reaching them hint at a much wider view of our minds: we have many more states and many more ways of achieving them. A multistate view of our minds emerges, and when our view of our minds changes, so does everything else. Although we will illustrate the usefulness of the "Multistate Theory" by specializing in psychedelics, always resting in the back of our minds is the knowledge that there is a vast horizon of other states behind our psychedelic foreground.

Chapter 8 introduces multistate theory, and chapter 9 explores cognition, intelligence, and the cognitive studies in light of its insights. When a new map of our minds is charted, it gives birth to new ways of thinking about things. In chapter 10 the multistate map will lead us to spot information that scholars often overlook, topics that deserve investigation in archaeology, anthropology, and history. They help fill out our psychedelic cultural background. With particular attention to events surrounding birth and prior to it, chapter 11 will sample some ways the perinatal level of Stanislav Grof's map of the mind enriches our framework for interpreting the psychorhetoric of war, a mescaline input into the philosophy and social commentary of existential philosopher Jean-Paul Sartre, and psychocriticism of the arts—in this case movies.

Speculating more freely, chapter 12 will pick up some leads from current biology and medicine and use them as stepping-stones to the idea that in the future human brains may surpass our own. Chapter 12, which calls such a possible superior brain a *neurosingularity,* may be along the line of psychedelic science fiction, but it illustrates that a complete study of any topic must go beyond the data given to challenge or confirm existing findings and to generate new lines of research.

8

Multistate Theory

APPS ARE TO DEVICES AS MINDBODY
STATES ARE TO MINDS

Imagine that you and I have a friend, Don, who has purchased a new computer or other electronic device, and we are talking with him about it.

YOU: What are you going to do with it?

DON: I'm going to play chess on it.

YOU: And download music and games?

DON: No, I'm going to play chess on it.

YOU: You can find maps and directions too.

DON: I said I'm going to play chess on it.

ME: You can do your taxes and banking and buy stuff too.

DON: No! I said I'm going to play chess.

ME: You can send messages too and pictures all around the
   world and for free too.

DON: NO! Didn't you hear me?! I said I'm going to play chess.
   That's what I got it for.

We recognize, of course, that our friend in this overdrawn example is vastly underutilizing his electronic information-processing system, and he could do much more with it if he wanted. Yet, we are all like Don. We vastly underuse an information-processing system many times more complex and with an enormous variety of programs. The system is our brain, and its programs are mindbody states. Like Don using only one program on his computer, most of us use only one program in our minds. Some people even insist the other programs don't exist, or if they do exist, they are useless.

The idea that our minds can produce and use many mindbody states and that some of them have uses is not new. In 1902 William James, father of psychology, expressed it in what is probably its best-known iteration.

> Some years ago I myself made some observations on this aspect of nitrous oxide intoxication, and reported them in print. One conclusion was forced upon my mind at that time, and my impression of its truth has ever since remained unshaken. It is that our normal waking consciousness, rational consciousness as we call it, is but one special type of consciousness, whilst all about it, parted from it by the filmiest of screens, there lie potential forms of consciousness entirely different. We may go through life without suspecting their existence; but apply the requisite stimulus, and at a touch they are there in all their completeness, definite types of mentality which probably somewhere have their field of application. No account of the universe in its totality can be final which leaves these other forms of consciousness quite disregarded. How to regard them is the question,—for they are so discontinuous with ordinary consciousness. (1902, 298)

Although this quotation is well known, its first sentence is often omitted. I suppose that is because it is naughty of James to have used a psychoactive drug to generate this insight. But thanks to psychedelics and other ways—both naughty and nice—of parting our filmy screens, James's idea has regained power and credibility.

BEYOND THE SINGLESTATE FALLACY

The "singlestate fallacy" is the erroneous assumption that all worthwhile abilities reside in our normal, awake mindbody state. Undermining this assumption, the chapters leading up to this one illustrate some values of mystical states. In 1969 Charles Tart, then a professor at the University of California at Davis, challenged psychology to fulfill its scientific task by including all the data in its field. "The most important obligation of any science is that its descriptive and theoretical language embrace all the phenomena of its subject matter; the data from [altered states of consciousness] cannot be ignored if we are to have a comprehensive psychology" (Tart 1969, 5).

Psychology's progress since then has been grudgingly slow, largely due to overfocusing on our default, awake state and relegating other states and their cognitive, emotional, perceptive, and behavioral processes to sideshow curiosities and odd anomalies. The title itself of a paper published by the American Psychological Association in 2004— *Varieties of Anomalous Experience: Examining the Scientific Evidence* (Cardena et al.)—betrays that organization's confusion in classifying altered-state experiences along with parapsychology and shoving both to the periphery of its field.

Although progress has been slow, Tart's injunction for psychology to include "all the data in its field" is picking up speed. Steadily, respectable amounts of multistate scientific knowledge and theory are accumulating. For example, in 2011 Cardena and Winkelman's two-volume set, *Altering Consciousness: Multidisciplinary Perspectives,* summarized the history, culture, and humanistic background as well as biological and psychological perspectives on altered states.

In contrast to the singlestate fallacy, multistate theory recognizes that the ability to produce and use a variety of mindbody states is a significant human trait. Far from discarding information about our ordinary state, multistate theory encompasses our ordinary state and especially values it as the mindbody state that has been most thoroughly studied. Existing singlestate findings are not discarded but contribute to a whole multistate map of our minds. Additionally, research on our usual, awake state illustrates methods and topics that the nascent studies of other states might emulate.

The shift to multistate theory produces three basic concepts: mindbody state, psychotechnologies, and residence.

MINDBODY STATE—THE PSYCHOGEOGRAPHY OF INNER STATES

Mindbody states are overall patterns of cognitive and bodily functioning at any one time. They are composed of body plus mind considered as one unified whole, such as the commonest states of wakefulness, sleeping, and dreaming. The word *mindbody* also avoids the ambiguity of the word *consciousness,* which is used in different ways in different disciplines and in common language. Confusion arises when people think that they are talking about the same thing when they use the same word. The primary uses of the word *consciousness* listed here, however, make it clear that the meanings are quite different, though at times overlapping.

Common language 1—*Consciousness* means awake and interacting normally with the environment: for example, "She is *conscious* now, but last night she was asleep," and "After being in a coma for three days, he is *conscious.*"

Common language 2—*Consciousness* refers to what one habitually thinks about, to what is typically "on one's mind" such as, "She has good ecological consciousness," or "His money occupies the center of his consciousness."

Politics and the social sciences—*Consciousness* means the thoughts and feelings one has constructed due to one's place in society, for example, *proletarian consciousness* or *women's consciousness.*

Philosophy—*Consciousness* refers to a self-reflective sense of "I": one thinks and can reflect on oneself and on one's thinking. In this case, the word *self-reflexiveness* would be more precise and avoid ambiguity.

Religion and spiritual discussions—*Consciousness* means level of spiritual development as in, "His mystical experience raised John's level of consciousness."

Psychology 1—*Consciousness* is the sequence of what one attends to second by second; what passes through one's mind becomes the *stream of consciousness.*

Psychology 2—Here *consciousness* refers to different overall patterns of mind and body functioning at any one time, as in Tart's "altered states of consciousness."

The final meaning listed here is the one I suggest replacing with *mindbody.* This will allow cognitive studies to avoid ambiguity and provides a way of specifying a particular pattern of mind plus body functioning at any one time.

Besides recognizing that many states are important, the mindbody concept points to a highly productive analogy for thinking about our minds: *apps are to devices as mindbody states are to minds.* Mindbody states function analogously to the way programs function in computers. This analogy does not mean that our brains are merely computers, but it implies that there may be many useful mindbody states just as there are many useful programs and apps. And just as we can write and install large numbers of electronic information-processing programs in our electronic devices, we can design and install a large number of bio-information-processing programs in our bodies.

As the next chapter on problem solving and enhanced intelligence shows, psychedelic mindbody programs, like computer programs, have their distinct applications. Both accept distinct types of input, process it their respective ways, and provide their characteristic outputs. Thus, the concept mindbody state alerts us to the full range of psychological and biological functioning.

PSYCHOTECHNOLOGIES—AGENTS OF TRANSFORMATION

The second major concept in multistate theory is *psychotechnology*. Usually when we think of technologies we think of electronic, biological, or mechanical technologies. Psychotechnologies are currently an under-recognized class of biotechnologies: techniques, methods, and treatments that produce states (install programs) that affect cognition, perception, emotion, and other psychological and biological processes. Among psychotechnologies are selected exercise routines, meditation, psychoactive plants and chemicals, yoga and the martial arts, sensory overload and sensory deprivation, hypnosis and receptive relaxation, chanting, dream work, breathing techniques, biofeedback and neurofeedback, transcranial magnetic stimulation, contemplative prayer, vision quests, drumming, and more. Each of these is not just one, lone psychotechnology, but a family of related techniques, such as the many types of meditation and contemplative prayer. A full map of the human mind needs to include all mindbody states, all their functions, and all the ways of achieving both.

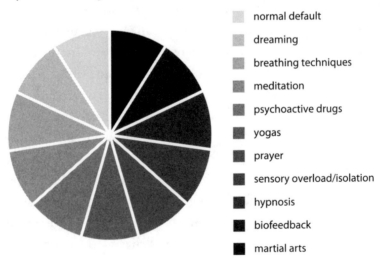

normal default

dreaming

breathing techniques

meditation

psychoactive drugs

yogas

prayer

sensory overload/isolation

hypnosis

biofeedback

martial arts

Figure 8.1. Diagram of an idea: a complete view of our minds must include all the mindbody states created by all psychotechnologies. The relative sizes of the slices have yet to be determined.

Along with economic globalization, the import and export of productive psychotechnologies is producing a globalization of ways to install an increasingly wide repertoire of mindbody programs. The list of psychoactive drugs reaches well into the hundreds. Similarly, lists of all kinds of meditation or of the many martial arts would quickly exceed dozens and perhaps even hundreds. I suppose a full census of psychotechnologies would reach into the thousands and remains a task to be accomplished.

Most important, if we are to have a complete map of the human mind, the cognitive sciences and related humanities need to study every topic they now investigate in our default mindbody state in all other states. The extensive field of psychotechnologies alerts us to a huge number of new research topics as well as methods and treatments available for this research. It unveils a vast future for cognitive studies, as all current questions are re-asked for every mindbody state—how every psychotechnology affects them. The concept of residence moves us in that direction.

RESIDENCE

The third major concept in the multistate theory is *residence*. Our mental and physical capacities reside within mindbody states; that is, mindbody states are the programs that express, or produce, outputs. To access the outputs, we first achieve the states that contain them. As we move from one state to another, we observe that some of our cognitive processes, perceptions, feelings, and abilities become stronger in some states and weaker in others; processes in one state have their analogs in others. This leads to an enormous question that blows the roof off nearly all the topics that psychologists, cognitive scientists, and humanists study: How does [insert a topic here] vary from mindbody state to mindbody state?

Applying the Central Multistate Question

How does/do _____ *vary from mindbody state to mindbody state?*

To sample the opportunities that the Central Multistate Question and its paradigm offer, try inserting the topics below into the question above. To invent additional hypotheses, questions, and intellectual agendas, insert your favorite topics.

cognition	consciousness	movement
meaning	learning	memory
language	aesthetics	theology
development	emotions	perception
performance	sensations	observation
values	identity	reason

As we move from one state to another, we may also discover new, different abilities—ones that do not exist in our ordinary state. Systematic exploration of all mindbody states and inventorying their resident abilities are two huge mind-mapping tasks that remain in the quest to fully describe the human mind.

Generally when we say a specific human behavior or experience is possible or impossible, we are implying but seldom acknowledging that we mean "in our ordinary awake state." Rare and unusual abilities and even some so-called impossible abilities and events may seem impossible to us because we have looked for them only in our default awake state. As we systematically examine other mindbody states, however, we are likely to find skills and abilities that don't reside in our ordinary state. In addition to alerting us to examine how an ability that we recognize, say, problem solving, varies from state to state, the concept of residence also alerts us to extend our vision of possible human functioning to abilities and events that do not reside in our default state.

WIDER THEORETICAL IMPLICATIONS

Multistate theory enhances a wider scientific endeavor. In addition to the "How does ____ vary" questions, mindbody states can be both independent and dependent variables. Vastly expanding the realm of scientific inquiry, all the families of psychotechnologies and all their family members become experimental treatments.

Experimental Humanities

Chapter 4, "The New Religious Era," gives some examples of how it is now possible to develop a new specialty of experimental religious studies. Philosophers can do similar experiments. How does mind vary from mindbody state to mindbody state? Do default state philosophical ideas hold in other mindbody states? What are we to make of these changes? Thanks to psychedelics and other psychotechnologies, philosophers can move beyond armchair speculation to study their topics experimentally too. Just as religion is moving beyond its word-anchored past, so can the humanities.

Volume 1 of Cardena and Winkelman's *Altering Consciousness* looks at consciousness (read *mindbody*) interests in history, cultural perspectives, philosophy, religion, literature, performance (including aesthetic and athletic), art, and music. The intersections of these fields with psychedelics and with other psychotechnologies open even more doors.

A Standard for Judging Empirical Findings and Theoretical Claims

Multistate Theory also provides a standard for judging the strength of empirical findings and generalizations. A general rule in research is: the more diverse a database, the stronger are the findings derived from it. While not falling into the trap of the Singlestate Fallacy, current research on meditation, hypnosis, dreams, and other mindbody states, including our default state, generally derive their data sets and theoretical generalizations from only one state. Identifying which findings hold across several states and which are state-specific will help design a more complex and complete map of cognition and other mental processes, including connections among states and similar and dissimilar structures.

Discovering Hidden Parameters

When we explore the human mind and try to educate it, we make assumptions about what our minds are and what they can do. We suppose some things can change while others remain constant. Changing or constant, the things we pay attention to are called *parameters;* they lead us to focus on some things and ignore others, especially those that we do not know exist.

Some parameters that are constant in singlestate psychology change in multistate psychology. An explicit example of this comes from Benny Shanon's work with ayahuasca. He identifies eleven parameters that singlestate mind studies miss. Three of the eleven he spots are 1) experiencing thoughts as not being one's own; 2) personal identification with whatever one is looking at, a sense of unity with the other; and 3) self-transcendence but with consciousness still maintained (2002). This is not to say that his discoveries are "real" in the ordinary singlestate sense, but they exist in the world of the mind, so a full study of the mind cannot exclude them. Our singlestate assumptions merely blind us to them. When we recognize that these can change, the ground underneath singlestate cognitive studies quakes. Chapter 14, "It Means Something Different to be Well Educated," contains Shanon's whole list. More important, his discoveries raise the broader question, "Will other mindbody explorers discover more shifting parameters?"

Research Studies

Typically a new theory reorganizes information, provides model experiments, new research directions, original questions, new variables, and innovative methods. By these criteria, the psychedelic wing of multistate theory certainly qualifies. Earlier chapters of this book have described some of these approaches, and later chapters will elaborate on others.

The thing to notice here is that information on multistate theory and psychedelic research combines many sources, giving a richness to its origins and credibility to its findings.

Biochemical studies—For nonspecialists, Perrine's *The Chemistry of Mind-altering Drugs* (1996) opens the door of exploration. In 2010 *The Pharmacology of LSD: A Critical Review* (Hintzen and Passie) reported on this aspect, including extensive references. The works of Alexander Shulgin combine the chemical and personal experience trails (1991, 1997, 2002, 2011).

Clinical case studies—LSD treatment has been used for a wide range of neuroses and psychoses, notably by Stanislav Grof. Passie's (1997) bibliography of 687 studies cross-references them by author, and the index lists them by type of study, condition treated, substance used, group or individual, and other treatment categories.

Clinical experiments—Grob's clinical experimentation with psilocybin at UCLA to reduce death anxiety, Mithoefer's study of MDMA (2007, 2011) as a treatment for post-traumatic stress disorder and similar studies reported elsewhere (www.maps.org) are the growing edge.

Experiential reports—Books on personal experiences (currently largely on ayahuasca experiences) are at flood tide. For calmer, more considered perspectives, I prefer Walsh and Grob's *Higher Wisdom* (2005) and Badiner's *Zig Zag Zen* (2002). They present reflective, in-depth phenomenological interviews.

General review of the literature—Although originally published in 1979, *Psychedelic Drugs Reconsidered,* by Lester Grinspoon and James B. Bakalar, at that time both on the faculty of Harvard Medical School, remains the best general review of the relevant literature. Subsequent paperback editions contain a magnificent forty-page annotated bibliography.

Medical perspectives—In 2007 Michael Winkelman, then an anthropologist at Arizona State University, and I compiled a two-volume set of essays whose title, *Psychedelic Medicine: New Evidence for Hallucinogenic Substances as Treatments,* describes the set. Updated works by some of the contributors appear in this book, and many of them have other works in progress.

Scientific laboratory—Psychedelic research designs are well exemplified by the Johns Hopkins laboratory nonclinical human experiments with psilocybin-occasioned mystical experiences (Griffiths et al. 2006, 2008, 2011).

Surveys—Hood's 1975 mysticism scale and Lerner and Lyvers's 2006 study of values and beliefs of psychedelic users illustrate survey methods.

The websites of the Multidisciplinary Association for Psychedelics Studies and the Heffter Research Institute offer helpful resources for keeping up to date on current research. The U.S. National Institutes of Health website (www.clinicaltrials.gov) lists clinical trials using hallucinogens (excluding cannabis and related compounds) of more than a dozen current trials. Although this and other online sources primarily report on the psychotherapeutic uses of psychedelics, hidden in them are reports on higher-level cognitive processes. Taken together, these publications and experiments alert us to the fact that psychedelics also offer experimental treatments for the study of abstraction, generalization, conceptualization, values, and beliefs.

DESIGNING AND INVENTING NEW COGNITIVE PROCESSES

Just as programmers can write a large number of new programs and apps for electronic devices, cognitive designers using psychotechnologies can compose a large number of programs for our minds. These programs and their applications are not limited to states we now know of; it may be possible for future cognitive scientists to invent new, hitherto unknown mindbody states containing new cognitive processes, possibly with their respective applications for human needs. This might be done by inventing new psychotechnologies, sequencing current or new psychotechnologies in innovative series, or by combining them into new recipes. The singlestate fallacy frowns on this possibility: multistate theory sees designing and creating new cognitive processes as a way to invent the future of the human mind.

SUMMARY

Multistate theory identifies areas needing systematic scientific investigation and provides ways to do so: the human mind is an experimental variable. Supported by psychedelic evidence, this theory (Roberts 1989, 2006) meets the requirements for a paradigm (Kuhn 1962), as listed below.

1. Includes previously excluded phenomena: Multistate theory includes observations from other mindbody states and their phenomena.

2. Posits new relationships among them: Multistate theory hypothesizes that the abilities of our usual awake state have analogs in other states and that additional abilities and cognitive processes exist in other states.

3. Introduces useful concepts: Multistate theory introduces the concepts of mindbody state, psychotechnologies, and residence.

4. Accepts and helps explain anomalies: Multistate theory helps explain ego transcendence and provides a strategy to investigate other-state phenomena, including so-called impossible events and those that are rare or unusual because they reside in other mindbody states.

5. Stimulates new research questions and agendas (new normal science): Multistate theory extends research to ask the question "How do/does ____ vary from mindbody state to mindbody state?" about all current topics in the cognitive sciences and humanities; it promotes the full characterization, exploration, and development of all known mindbody states plus the possible construction of new ones.

6. Provides new variables, treatments, and methodologies: Multistate theory provides psychotechnologies as research treatments and mindbody states as both independent and dependent variables.

7. Strengthens professional preparation: Multistate theory proposes to strengthen the professional education of cognitive scientists and other scholars to include the study of the full range of cognitive processes, and proposes experimentation in religious studies and other disciplines.

8. Includes a group of professionals who use this paradigm: Although not explicitly using multistate theory, the work of researchers cited in this book and elsewhere—their assumptions, models, independent and dependent variables, instruments, and findings—fit snugly within multistate theory.

Multistate theory offers prospects of increased cognitive flexibility and a freer flow of ideas; however, just as with our ordinary default state, not all these ideas will be worthwhile. They will also have to be tested and evaluated. From a multistate perspective, one of the most informative intellectual activities you can experience is the exploration of mindbody states. How to do this provides challenging opportunities for bright minds now and in the future.

9

Enhancing Cognition, Boosting Intelligence, Expanding Cognitive Studies

Current research offers some tantalizing support for claims that psychedelics can be used to enhance cognition, improve intelligence, and strengthen cognitive studies.

COGNITIVE ENHANCEMENT

Experimental evidence of psychedelic cognitive enhancement comes from studies of practical problem solving, abstract concepts, and psychotherapy.

The Sleeping Giant of Psychedelics' Future—
Innovative Problem Solving

A significant instance of problem solving resulted in a Nobel Prize for Kary Mullis. Until the invention of the polymerase chain reaction (PCR), a common problem in biology was that biological samples were often too small to analyze, but Mullis solved that and won a Nobel Prize. He described how LSD aided him in doing so.

> PCR's another place where I was down there with the molecules when I discovered it and I wasn't stoned on LSD, but my mind by then had learned how to get down there. I could sit on a DNA molecule and watch the [indistinct] go by. . . . I've learned that partially I would think, and this is again my opinion, through psychedelic drugs . . . if I had not taken LSD ever would I have still been in PCR? I don't know, I doubt it, I seriously doubt it. (Mullis 1998; "Horizon: Psychedelic Science" 1997)

From the point of view of psychedelic cognitive studies, Mullis's example is noteworthy because he did not have his insight while taking psychedelics but instead used psychedelics to increase his ability to visualize, then transferred that cognitive skill back to his ordinary mindbody state. This confirms the idea that some skills learned in one state can be transferred to another. Transference and nontransference between mindbody states is itself a cognitive process that deserves study—learning to remember dreams, for example. Learning to increase this flow, if it is possible, would increase access to stores of information and possibly to new cognitive skills.

Unlike Mullis's experience of transferring a skill back to his ordinary state, most instances of psychedelic problem solving occur while the person's cognitive processes are psychedelically augmented. This is most clearly illustrated by "Psychedelic Agents in Creative Problem Solving: A Pilot Study," by Willis Harman, a professor of engineering economic systems, and a team of researchers at Stanford Research Institute. Working with twenty-seven men who were "engaged in various professional occupations, i.e., engineers, physicists, mathematicians, architects, a furniture designer, and a commercial artist and had a total of 44 professional problems they wanted to work on," the Stanford Research Institute team divided them into groups of three or four and gave them 200 milligrams of mescaline, followed by a quiet period of listening to music. Then they had snacks and discussed their problems with their group. Following this they spent three or four hours working alone on their problems. As a result of psychedelic enhancement, the practical results were impressive.

Pragmatic Utility of Solutions. The practical value of obtained solutions is a check against subjective reports of accomplishment which might be attributable to temporary euphoria. The nature of these solutions was varied; they included: (1) a new approach to the design of a vibratory microtome, (2) a commercial building design accepted by client, (3) space probe experiments devised to measure solar properties, (4) design of a linear electron accelerator beam-steering device, (5) engineering improvement to magnetic tape recorder, (6) a chair design modeled and accepted by manufacturer, (7) a letterhead design approved by customer, (8) a mathematical theorem regarding NOR-gate circuits, (9) completion of a furniture line design, (10) a new conceptual model of a photon which was found useful, and (11) design of a private dwelling approved by the client. (Fadiman 2011, 132)

James Fadiman, one of the coauthors of this study, describes it and other psychedelic approaches to problem solving in his 2011 book *The Psychedelic Explorer's Guide*. His valuable descriptions of their process as seen by an investigator-insider and quotations from the problem solvers themselves draw attention to this sleeping giant of psychedelics' future—practical problem solving. It is time for researchers to awaken this giant and for federal agencies and local institutional review boards to move forward and encourage creative invention.

It is a widely known "inside secret" that psychedelics also contributed to the rapid innovation and growth of the personal computer industry (Markoff 2006), and probably the greatest monetary payoff from using psychedelics occurred when the problem of a little start-up software company vying with other start-ups for the eyes of potential customers was solved.

The big quandary for software companies was getting into the market place, finding shelf space. But there was a new way of doing that I thought of called "shareware," and I think the concept was very unusual, and I think the concept came to some extent from my psychedelic experience. . . . So that worked. It worked pretty well. (Wallace 1997)

Bob Wallace's idea was to give away programs and ask people to pay whatever they could and wanted to. Because they were free, thousands of people started using them, and this helped his little, unknown start-up company grab market share so that eventually it could charge for its products and begin to turn a profit: micrograms for Microsoft.

Experimental Studies of Abstract Concepts

Much research in the cognitive sciences has to do with memorizing things not worth memorizing, solving silly puzzles, and other unrealistic tasks that lend themselves to clean laboratory research designs but have little relevance in life. This barrier was broken and cognitive studies advanced to higher level thinking thanks to psilocybin. In 2006 and 2008, experiments showed that psychedelics can extend cognitive studies to topics that are important in people's lives but were previously beyond experimentation—meaningfulness and significance among others (Griffiths et al. 2006, 2008, 2011).

In previous chapters we've looked at the implications of these experiments for values and religion; here our concern is their implications for higher level cognitive psychology. They found, "at 2 months, the volunteers rated the psilocybin experiences as having substantial personal meaning and spiritual significance and attributed to the experience sustained positive changes in attitudes and behavior consistent with changes rated by community observers" (Griffiths et al. 2006, 268). To account for the possibility that their volunteers might overrate their own behavior, the Hopkins team interviewed friends and close family members to see if they noticed any changes, which they confirmed. This experiment illustrates how psychedelics can advance experimental studies far beyond trivial attention span and boring digit-memory tasks to the high level abstractions that give meaning to people's lives.

Three written comments express the essence of the participants' experiences.

- The understanding that in the eyes of God—all people . . . were all equally important and equally loved by God. I have had other transcendent experiences, however, this one was important because it reminded and comforted me that God is truly and unconditionally loving and present.

- Freedom from every conceivable thing including time, space, relationships, self, etc. . . . It was as if the embodied "me" experienced ultimate transcendence—even of myself.

- A non-self self held/suspended in an almost tactile field of light. (629)

These three samples of enhanced spiritual cognition demonstrate that psychedelics provide a breakthrough for the cognitive sciences: instead of being limited to surveys, random self-reports, and lightly grounded speculation about higher level cognitive processes such as meaningfulness, sacredness, and significance, psychedelics enhance cognitive sciences with an experimental method of investigating these and similar high-level, abstract conceptualizations.

Experimental Religious Studies

With its heavy reliance on words, beliefs, and text, current religion, of course, is heavily cognitive, so it provides another avenue for advancing cognitive studies. "Experimental religious studies" sounds impossible, but thanks to psychedelics it isn't. The findings of Griffiths's group and other reports illustrate one way to use psychedelics to study higher-level abstractions, in this case religious ones.

As mentioned earlier, the best example of the long-term influence of psychedelics on thinking is Rick Doblin's 2001 study "Pahnke's Good Friday Experiment: A Long-term Follow-up and Methodological Critique." Doblin is the founding executive director of the Multidisciplinary Association for Psychedelic Studies. Its website is one of the richest of the psychedelic Internet domains. MAPS is primarily interested in psychotherapy, but reading its publications and website from a cognitive perspective is like stumbling into a great hidden treasure. Doblin's follow-up study documenting the effects of psilocybin given to seminarians a quarter of a century earlier speaks to the power of psychedelics as experimental treatments and to mystical experiences as experimental variables. I look forward to reading a "Journal of Experiential Religion."

Cognitive Aspects of Psychedelic Psychotherapy

Psychedelic psychotherapy is more than a treatment. It has implications beyond health; it provides clues to how our minds work. How does thinking change during successful psychotherapy, such as when psilocybin is used to reframe death anxiety in the work of Charles Grob and his coresearcher Alicia Danforth, or MDMA-assisted psychotherapy is used to reduce post-traumatic stress disorder in patients who have been intractable to other treatments, as in the work of South Carolina psychiatrist Michael Mithoefer?* Other clinical leads suggest treating cluster headaches, obsessive-compulsive disorder, neuroses and psychoses, depression, alcoholism, and addiction.

Except for cluster headaches, these cures are usually correlated with mystical experiences. Cognitively, what phenomenological shifts occur during mystical experiences, with the power to reframe thoughts, emotions, and identity so much that they apparently often cure death anxiety, post-traumatic stress disorder, and addictions and alcoholism? Hood's mysticism scale and similar measures of mystical experience may provide clues. In his 1996 "The Facilitation of Religious Experience," Hood summarizes the evidence that psychedelics often produce mystical experiences, and in his 2006 "The Common Core Thesis in the Study of Mysticism," he compares phenomenologically derived and empirically derived models of mystical experience. For cognitive scientists who want to study higher order processes experimentally, the items in Hood's scale may be clues to how to study this type of cognitive reframing.

---

*It is important to keep in mind that in both these clinical experiments the drugs were used as adjuncts to psychotherapy, not alone as a pharmacological study. This should be a warning against self-prescribing: it is the combination of the drug and psychotherapy that works. Psychedelic adjuncts to psychotherapy alone will not give the same results.

IMPROVING INTELLIGENCE

Howard Gardner, best known for his theory of multiple intelligences, defines *intelligence* as "the ability to solve problems or produce goods of value to society" (1983). The instances cited above meet his standard for intelligence. Unfortunately, Gardner, like other scholars, defines and describes intelligence as it exists only in our ordinary, default mindbody state. A full view of intelligence would include the skillful use of all states. Recognizing that varieties of intelligence exist in states other than our usual awake state raises the question of whether other cognitive processes have their analogs in other mindbody states too, suggesting a future for multistate cognitive science—researching the question, "How does cognition vary from mindbody state to mindbody state?"

In *The Triarchic Mind,* Robert Sternberg suggests another criterion for intelligence, defining it as "mental self-management" (1988). By that standard, someone who can access a large collection of information-processing programs and their resident abilities is more intelligent than someone with a smaller repertoire. Kary Mullis's learning to strengthen his visualization capacity and transfer it to his usual state is an example. What about someone who is highly skilled at selecting mindbody states, achieving them, and using their resident abilities? Because selecting mindbody states is an executive function prior to the use of specific states, the word *metaintelligence* may be useful when discussing this kind of intelligence.

ENRICHING COGNITIVE STUDIES

Not only can cognitive science investigate cognitive enhancement, but by surpassing its current boundaries it can also accelerate the pace of its own scientific progress. Identifying and characterizing cognitive processes (and other processes) that exist in all mindbody states will demand new talents for skilled psychologists, phenomenologists, and neuropsychologists. In order to develop this agenda, a new generation of researchers needs to become comfortable studying these states both objectively and subjectively.

Cognitively, psychotechnologies are ways of installing information-processing programs in our minds. Among the many possibilities, psychedelics illustrate a vast multistate frontier for the future of cognitive studies, one in which mindbody states are sometimes "independent variables"—the things that experimenters change—and sometimes "dependent variables"—the things that change as a result. To put it another way: independent variables are the inputs and dependent variables are the outputs. For example, in the Johns Hopkins studies, psilocybin was the independent variable, and people's experiences were the dependent ones.

Examples include the clinical laboratory experiments we have already looked at in earlier chapters such as those by Griffiths, Grob, Mithoefer, and Grof. Hood's mysticism scale and Lerner and Lyvers's study of values and beliefs of psychedelic users illustrate survey methods. Walsh and Grob's 2005 *Higher Wisdom* and Badiner's 2008 *Zig Zag Zen* present in-depth phenomenological interviews. Nichols and Chemel connect chemistry and religious cognition in their article 2006 "The Neuropharmacology of Religious Experience." An Internet search of clinical trials using hallucinogens (excluding cannabis and related compounds) locates more than a dozen current trials, while the MAPS website keeps readers up-to-date on completed, current, and planned research.

Perhaps the most curious and exciting prospect psychedelics offer is their impact on humanistic and religious concepts such as meaningfulness, significance, portentousness, values, transcendence, self-concept, aesthetic perception, identity, beliefs, and sacredness. These abstractions form the vitals of humanistic studies, but until psychedelics, they have been hard to study in experiments. The provocative psychedelic studies throughout this book indicate that these abstractions may become dependent variables when mindbody states are the independent variables.

Consilience

In 1998 biologist Edward O. Wilson, author of two Pulitzer Prize–winning books and recipient of other honors and awards, challenged the scientific community to build a multidisciplinary cognitive structure that integrates all branches of knowledge. He called his book and the project *Consilience*. Psychedelics are a natural for this major league intellectual project. They are naturally interdisciplinary. They link topics from the neurochemistry of our brains to Greek mythology and film criticism. As the Griffiths et al. studies of the effects of psilocybin on personal meaningfulness and sacredness exemplify, psychedelics provide one way to overcome the problem of integrating different lines of inquiry into a multilayered scaffolding of empirical evidence.

How do the chemical, biological, psychological, cognitive, and social levels influence each other? With psychedelics questions such as "How do biochemical changes affect beliefs?" are open to experimentation. Conversely, researchers can experimentally examine the question "How do someone's beliefs and cognitive expectations influence the outcomes of biochemical experimental treatments?" By providing models for independent variables on one level and dependent variables on others, meditation, psychedelics, and other mindbody psychotechnologies provide ready-made roads to advance the consilience project.

Wilson recognized this. "Shamans preside over the taking of hallucinogenic drugs and interpret the meaning of the serpents and other apparitions that subsequently emerge" (1998, 72). He reports, "[The shaman's] drug of choice, widely used in the communities of the Rio Ucayali region, is ayahuasca [pronounced eye-uh-WAHS-ska], extracted from the jungle vine *Banisteriopsis*." Illustrating consilience, he follows this with, "The sacred plants, which have been analyzed by chemists, are no longer mysterious. Their juices are laced with neuromodulators that in large oral doses produce a state of excitation, delirium, and vision" (73). Wilson recognized that chemical input yields cognitive output, yet another instance of the chemical-cognitive relationship that most of the researchers mentioned above have implicitly noted.

Discovering Hidden Parameters of the Mind

Although the mentioned studies have implications for the cognitive sciences, they were not expressly designed to do so. Shanon's *The Antipodes of the Mind: Charting the Phenomenology of the Ayahuasca Experience* intentionally hybridizes cognitive psychology and psychedelics.

> Not only can a cognitive-psychological analysis make a crucial contribution to the study of Ayahuasca, the converse is also the case—the study of Ayahuasca may have implications of import to our general understanding of the working of the human mind. Ayahuasca (along with other mind-altering substances) expands the horizons of psychology and reveals new, hitherto unknown territories of the mind. Thus the study of Ayahuasca presents new data pertaining to human consciousness, and thus new issues for investigation, new ways to look at things, new questions, and perhaps even new answers. (2002, 37)

Shanon claims that one contribution of studying nonordinary mindbody states is "rendering the parameters of the cognitive system apparent and revealing the various possible values these parameters may take" (196). Will additional explorations into other mindbody states using other psychotechnologies discover still more of cognition's hidden parameters? Many assumptions that singlestate cognitive psychologists make about "givens" are based on data only or predominantly from our usual awake state. Some of their supposedly stable assumptions are really unrecognized variables, taking on other values in other states. By illustrating how the cognitive sciences and psychedelics can inform each other, his work models an enhanced multistate cognitive science.

The Omitted Evidence

Current professional discussions of cognitive enhancement (e.g., the 2008 Committee on Military and Intelligence Methodology for Emergent Neurophysiological and Cognitive/Neural Science Research in the Next Two Decades) and articles in consumer periodicals (Greely et al. 2008; Greely 2009; Talbot 2009) omit the strongest evidence. These omissions all have to do with psychedelics. While the contribution of psychedelics to music (Bromell 2000), art (Masters and Huston

1968; Johnson 2011), religion (Smith 2000; Roberts 2012), medicine (Winkelman and Roberts 2007), and psychotherapy are becoming recognized, recognition of their contributions to cognitive enhancement lags. Whether this omission is due to a simple lack of information or scientists' and scholars' fear for their careers by touching a taboo topic is hard to say; it is probably some of both.

Whatever the reason, the scientific climate is changing, as the title of Morris's 2008 editorial in *The Lancet* put it, "Research on Psychedelics Moves into the Mainstream" (1,491). It is time for the cognitive studies to wake up. Dormant leads from the 1950s to the 1970s are being picked up now, and four decades of updated research methods in the neurosciences are moving this frontier forward again. Society benefits from intellectual work. If chemicals make that work more efficient, insightful, and creative, isn't it a professional duty for intellectuals to work as well as they can by using chemical cognitive enhancers?

SUMMARY

As important as psychedelics are for enhancing cognition, strengthening intelligence, and fulfilling cognitive studies, the psychedelic group is only one group of mindbody techniques among others. Meditation, biofeedback and neurofeedback, the martial arts, yoga, breathing techniques, contemplative prayer, and selected exercise routines, rites of passage, and vision quests are other ways of producing a fuller range of mindbody states. They deserve careful attention too. Chapters parallel to this one could be written for each of them and for others.

10

New Intellectual Endeavors

How do psychedelics help us think differently about our lives and the world? The ideas that psychedelics generate lead to new topics. When they are blended into existing disciplines, they often open up surprising insights and create a rich intellectual geography. There is much too much scholarly labor being done on these topics for us to present a full picture; here we are taking only a visitor's quick snapshots of the much larger and more detailed multistate landscape of ideas. This chapter samples contributions from anthropology, archaeology, and history, then ends with some curious psychedelic mind candies.

THE GREAT FLOW OF MULTISTATE IDEAS

All the disciplines diagrammed in chapter 1 and all the psychotechnologies mentioned in chapter 8 flow into the mindbody intellectual revolution. Farther upstream along the tributaries are their respective smaller rivers, streams, creeks, and brooks—meditation ponds, martial arts streams, yoga flows, and an assortment of breathing brooks. In this book we explore some branches of the psychedelic tributary.

Anthropology and the Natural Plant Tributary
Eliade Updated
Before we go further, a lingering error needs to be addressed. Famed

anthropologist of religion Mircea Eliade originally considered the use of psychoactive plants as a degenerative form of shamanism. But as he learned of new discoveries on this topic, he changed his mind. Unfortunately, people unfamiliar with his revised views still cling to the famous man's original words. In their 1994 book *Ancient Traditions,* Gary Seaman and Jane Day report on Eliade's later informed opinions.

> I should note that in the last years of [Eliade's] productive life, although unable to amend his views in a new, revised edition of *Shamanism,* he had discarded his view of the use of hallucinogenic plants as "degeneration" of the shamanic techniques of ecstasy. The work done by ethnobotanists and ethnographers on the vast complex of shamanic uses of sacred plants in the Americas, the emerging philological evidence for widespread and very ancient use of the fly-agaric mushroom in Europe, and, finally, the new radiocarbon dates from the American Southwest, he told me not long before his death, had convinced him that we were indeed dealing with an archaic phenomenon and that there was no phenomenological difference between the techniques of ecstasy, whether "spontaneous" or triggered by the chemistry of sacred plants. Another element that entered into his reconsideration, he said, was the recognition that the Arctic was settled relatively late in Siberian prehistory. Arctic forms of shamanism could thus no longer be held to be ancestral to shamanism in the more temperate regions of northeastern Asia. None of this is meant to suggest that the ecstatic trance experience is dependent upon ingestion of a particular ritual intoxicant. There are large areas in which visions and the ecstatic trance are highly valued and even considered essential but in which no psychoactive substances are employed for this purpose. (22)

The Anthropology of Consciousness

Giving chronological depth and cultural scope to psychedelic studies, the anthropology of consciousness (Society for the Anthropology of

Consciousness) and archaeology are giving broad backgrounds to the mindbody revolution, setting it within the huge flow of human history going back thousands of years and stretching geographically around the world. In her 1973 book *Religion, Altered States of Consciousness, and Social Change,* anthropologist Erica Bourguignon considers humanity's desire to change consciousness. She rhetorically asks herself, "[A]re we dealing with a major aspect of human behavior that has significant impact on the functioning of human societies?" She answers, ". . . of a sample of 488 societies, in all parts of the world, for which we have analyzed the relevant ethnographic literature, 437, or 90%, are reported to have one or more institutionalized, culturally patterned forms of altered states of consciousness" (9). Not all of these are psychoactive plants of course, but her observation embeds alterations in mindbody states in a solid cultural perspective.

This illustrates anthropologists' growing interest in mindbody topics. Now when they study cultures, they are likely to ask:

- What psychotechnologies does this culture use?
- What mindbody states do they produce?
- How do they use the states?
- How do they understand them?

These mindbody questions are popping up across the scholarly and scientific landscape. The anthropology of consciousness and its subspecialty of psychedelic anthropology are so rich and complex it is hard to select a few samples. Among my favorites are the well-illustrated Schultes and Hofmann's 1992 *Plants of the Gods* in which they globally map psychoactive plants. In most cases psychoactive plants are eaten as found or simply processed, say, as a tea or smoked. Judging from current anthropological studies, the anthropological river is likely to report that cultures attribute some sort of spiritual force to the plants. In *The Antipodes of the Mind* (2002), Benny Shanon hybridizes cognitive psychology and anthropology for their mutual benefit. The chapter "Psychedelic Drugs in Pre-industrial Society" from Grinspoon and Bakalar's 1979 *Psychedelic Drugs*

Reconsidered reviews and compiles writings on psychedelics. Harner's 1973 classic anthology, *Hallucinogens and Shamanism,* collects his own more detailed observations along with those of nine other contributors. These and a hundred or more other books enrich the mindbody river with cross-cultural complexity.

The tributary of native plant history is not just a dry arroyo or cultural oddity but continues to flow into the psychedelic river. Anthropologists are still documenting how different contemporary cultures use psychoactive plants, both psychedelic and others, and some of these or information about them are being imported into Western scholarship and enriching it—streams of information about ayahuasca, ibogaine, and peyote, for instance.

Archaeology: Digging Up the Far Past

Archaeologists provide another tributary. Among other findings, they have unearthed remains of psychoactive plants in Neanderthal graves stretching as far back as 50,000 years ago, perhaps longer in current Shanidar, Iraq.

> The last of the six main plants is woody horsetail (*Ephedra*), which has a long history of use in Asian and other medical practices. It was once thought that *Ephedra* was the fabled soma of the ancient Indians, a psychoactive plant consumed by priests during their rituals. It is not a suitable candidate as it has amphetamine-like stimulant effects rather than the hallucinogenic properties attributed to *soma*. Nevertheless, it is known from archaeological sites in prehistoric Central Asia to have been consumed with more potent substances, such as opium and cannabis. Its more widespread use is as a remedy used to treat coughs and respiratory disorders, and in modern times extracts of it have been used to treat asthma. (Rudgley 1999, 216)

Drawing on observations from his own psychedelic trip to Neolithic passage tombs in Western Europe in *The Long Trip: A Prehistory of*

Psychedelia, Paul Devereux points out, "our modern culture stands out in the long record of human history because of its difficulty in accepting in an orderly and integrated way the role of natural substances" (1997, ix).

Rudgley's *Essential Substances: A Cultural History of Intoxicants in Society* starts with stone age alchemy and visits Native Americans' use of peyote and possibly other psychoactive plants; as foreword writer William Emboden said, "It is a profound and much-needed interpretation of how society has been shaped by intoxicants" (Rudgley 1997, iii).

History: No! Not the Ancient Greeks and Romans!

Could the birth of Western culture contain an expression of psychoactive plants? What a horrifying thought! One of my personally favorite books answers "yes" and illustrates the natural plant influences in classical Greece and adjacent cultural areas. In *The Apples of Apollo* (2001), Carl Ruck, a professor of classics at Boston University with a specialty in the botany of the ancient Near East, the late Blaise D. Staples, Ph.D., who wrote on ancient Greek literature and culture, and Clark Heinrich, who wrote *Magic Mushrooms in Religion and Alchemy,* provide extensive evidence that Christianity, Judaism, and Hellenistic mystery cults all had roots in "a sacred ethnopharmacology, with traditions going back to earlier ages of the ancient world" (2002).

In the extensively footnoted and referenced *Apples,* Ruck, Staples, and Heirich mine Greek myths for hidden references to mushrooms and other psychoactive plants. They point out the frequently missed myco-origins of the early Greek city of Mycenae, located because its founder, Perseus, found a mushroom there. In the chapter "Jason, the Drug Man" they spot the shamanism of early Greece as a significant root of Western culture. "The fleece, apples, and serpents—represent the fly-agaric mushroom" (118). When fly-agaric mushroom caps are carefully dried, they "turn a metallic golden-orange color" so that the Argo's cruise was to pick up a cargo of "golden fleece" (118). In the chapter "Jesus, the Drug Man," the authors trace plant-stage sources of

Christianity. This is a chapter that is sure to raise the self-righteous ire of bibliolaters and, at the same time, challenge serious scholars of Christianity's history not to neglect these possible origins.

What happens when a master's student in biology switches fields and earns another master's and a Ph.D. in Classics? D. C. A. Hillman's biological perspective directed his attention to the plants of ancient Greece and Rome, and he wrote a dissertation that included the uses of psychoactive plants—both medicinal and recreational—in ancient Rome. Because scholars appreciate fresh insights into their fields of study and especially value perspectives that shine a light into previously neglected dark corners, his dissertation examination committee should have been delighted with Hillman's novel insights. However, as he relates:

> The choice was simple. Take out the chapter on the ancient world's recreational drug use, and any reference to narcotics in the rest of the dissertation. . . . After all, the most vocal member of my committee, the head of the department, had refuted my conclusion that the Romans used recreational drugs with the seemingly nonacademic response, "They just wouldn't do such a thing." After years of research, the best that academia had to offer was an anachronistic presupposition: We think drugs are bad, so why wouldn't they? (2008, 2)

In *The Chemical Muse*, D. C. A. Hillman develops the idea that psychoactive plants played a significant role in the dawn of Western civilization and its early hours. Among the celebrants of the rites of ancient Eleusis—including kykeon, the apparently ergotized eucharist—were Aristotle, Sophocles, Plato, Aeschylus, Pindar, Cicero, and several Roman emperors. But Hillman's idea was not well received. "Despite the volume of ancient literature concerned with the preparation and administration of potent botanicals, few academicians bothered to familiarize themselves with the ins and outs of drug use in antiquity" (218).

The History of Psychedelics

Everything has its history and many psychedelic books start out with a chapter that summarizes these drugs' history; there is a good flock of books that are actually histories of psychedelics. In my class, I use Jay Stevens's *Storming Heaven: LSD and the American Dream* (1987). Previously, I used *Acid Dreams: The Complete Social History of LSD: The CIA, the Sixties, and Beyond* (Lee and Shlain 1994). Of course, the book does not live up to its extravagant subtitle, but it is entertaining to read about the CIA's and Army's (mis)uses, which included running whorehouses. It's nice to know that taxpayers' money went for some good use. Sessa's *The Psychedelic Renaissance* updates the historical perspective to 2012. A British psychiatrist, he includes significant historical figures such as Roland Sandison, who pioneered early psychedelic psychiatry in England.

Psychedelic Psychiatry: LSD from Clinic to Campus by Erica Dyck (2008) and *Albion Dreaming* by Andy Roberts (2008) are also especially informative because they fill in gaps that are often missed by American historians. Dyck includes many of the significant Canadian details and people including Humphry Osmond, who coined the word *psychedelic;* she also found archival papers tucked away in repositories in the Prairie Provinces. Among Roberts's finds is the fact that LSD "arrived" in America when Viennese doctor Otto Kauders held a conference at Boston Psychiatric Hospital in 1949, and this transatlantic gem: "Research psychiatrist Max Rinkel, a delegate to the conference, immediately ordered some LSD from Sandoz and gave a 100 [microgram] dose to his enthusiastic colleague Dr. Robert Hyde, who became the first person on American soil to have the LSD experience" (Roberts 2008, 17).

AMUSES-TÊTES

Some of the things I most enjoy about studying psychedelics are the delightful unexpected oddities that pop up. I hope, and expect, more will appear from time to time. Here are a few of my favorites.

Geology + Toxicology

Digging into psychedelic research unearths some surprising gems in surprising disciplines, such as one recorded in an article in the *Journal of Clinical Toxicology*, "The Delphic Oracle: A Multidisciplinary Defense of the Gaseous Vent Theory" (Spiller et al. 2002). It was preceded by an article in the journal *Geology*, an unlikely read for psychedelic scholars. However, in 2001 it printed "New Evidence for the Geological Origins of the Ancient Delphic Oracle (Greece)" (de Boer et al.). Then in 2003 *Scientific American* published "Questioning the Delphic Oracle" (Hale et al.). In 2008 the *Journal of the Geological Society* elaborated with "Scent of a Myth: Tectonics, Geochemistry and Geomythology at Delphi (Greece)" (Piccardi et al.). As its subtitle indicates, it blends tectonics, chemistry, mythology, and archaeology. What an astounding example of how multistate theory can encourage different disciplines to support each other!

Taken together, the articles suggest that the oracles at ancient Delphi may have inhaled psychoactive fumes to obtain the mindbody states that produced their prognostications. At that time two geological faults crossed under the oracle's chamber. A rock layer contained bituminous limestone. When this layer became hot under pressure caused by fault movement, the rocks released ethylene gas, which got picked up by hot springs and taken to the surface. In a somewhat enclosed room and seated on a stool above a spring, the oracle known as the Pythia inhaled the gases and spoke her sayings. Over the years, however, the flow was cut off by several earthquakes and a buildup of mineral deposits that plugged the spring. While enriching our understanding of these aspects of ancient Roman and Greek history, this discovery also adds a previously unknown psychotechnology . . . natural psychoactive gas carried by a natural hot water spring.

A Halloween Story

Why were the witchcraft trials held in Salem, Massachusetts, and in eight other nearby Essex County villages? Why also in Fairfield, Connecticut? And why in 1692? It had been forty-seven years since the previous epidemic of witchcraft persecution in England. Why didn't it happen in other New England counties? What specifically triggered these events? Why did similar events take place in Europe centuries earlier? Why there, and why then? Combining clues from history, meteorology, agriculture, and medicine (actually, the lack of good medicine), Linnda Caporael found ergot, a fungus that grows on some cereal grains and grasses, to be the culprit in colonial Salem (1976), and now-retired University of Maryland historian Mary Matossian points the guilty finger at ergot several times in the history of Western Europe as well (1989).

Like many fungi and molds, ergot thrives in damp and cold places. Finding a diary that reported the daily weather, Caporael found this weather in Salem. Matossian finds time after time when ergot-prone weather preceded panics of witchcraft throughout the history of Western Europe and Russia. "A person suffering from ergotism may be prone to hallucinations, spasms, and twitches, and in the villages of Europe, these symptoms were attributed to witchcraft" (67). These seldom occurred in drier regions and where dairy foods rather than grains were the main diet. While the Salem witchcraft trials are largely interpreted as an epidemic of social panic in suggestible people, its origin stems clearly from ergotism. Cows also acted strangely and died, and it is hard to imagine cows getting caught up in a runaway social panic. Both cows and people ate the local grain, and both acted strangely. In my class meeting nearest Halloween, I show the PBS video *Witches Curse*, which follows the ergot theme from Salem back to an ancient bog burial in today's Denmark and a 1950s case of ergot poisoning in the village Pont Saint Esprit in France.

Urology!

A peculiarity of psychoactive mushrooms is that when they are excreted in urine, the urine is similarly psychoactive. A supposed way to identify a witch is to have her urinate on bread, then feed the bread to a dog. If the dog shows signs of being bewitched, then the investigators have found the culprit. This happened in Salem, and a dog in France met a similar fate. (I wonder what ancient medical doctor discovered this and how.) Bringing the urine story up to date, an empirically minded professional friend reports:

> We looked at each other and laughed nervously, and retired to opposite corners of the room where we filled our respective containers. . . . [I]t was glowing with a fiery orange cast. Since we were about to drink it we first smelled it to see what we were in for and were surprised at its pleasant odour, or rather, its fragrance. . . .
>
> Even before we drank, we were feeling good. Very good. Extremely good. But within minutes after drinking something amazing started to happen. My body began to feel very light, as though I weighed almost nothing. It felt as if the molecules that comprised my body were separating and allowing air to pass through, or that I could feel the space between atoms. I became aware of tremendous energy at my feet that rose up through my body in wave after wave. "Feeling good" was rapidly changing into the most blissful feelings I had ever experienced. I looked at Michael and he was radiant, truly radiant. We started laughing and exclaiming in disbelief as the bliss kept increasing. My mind and entire body were in the throes of a kind of meta-orgasm that wouldn't stop—not that I wanted it to. (Heinrich 2002, 193)

One can only admire Heinrich's dedication to the sacrifices one must sometimes make for empirical knowledge. I wonder how institutional review boards would react to proposals to replicate this research and what would be used as a control substance. Reindeer in northern Scandinavia and Siberia know how to get high; they follow shamans who eat psychoactive mushrooms in order to eat their yellow snow, and that brings us to zoology.

Zoology

Where did the idea of Santa's flying reindeer come from? Maybe we have the answer. Would it not make more sense to have flying geese, eagles, or other birds, even seagulls? In my class a favorite among the students' self-selected books is *Animals and Psychedelics* (2000). Giorgio Samorini, an Italian scholar specializing in psychoactive plants, reports that squirrels, chipmunks, goats, and caribou also go out of their way to eat *amanita muscaria* mushrooms and go out of their minds when they do (38–42). Irresponsible drug-induced behavior is not the prerogative of humans. When caribou come across psychedelic mushrooms during their long migration, Samorini reports, the females will literally step out of line and do shrooms. They abandon their calves and run around shaking their heads and swinging hindquarters. They and their calves become easy prey for wolves.

Going beyond psychedelics, *Animals and Psychedelics* describes cows crazed on locoweed, elephants drunk on fermented fruit to the point they overreact to unusual noises. In a similar manner to young adult human males having binge drinking contests, "groups of elephants appear to compete over the fruits, each of them trying to eat the most fruit in the shortest time possible" (28). Other mammals, birds, and even insects seem to have a built-in desire for psychoactive plants. Why?

In his 1989 book *Intoxication,* Ronald Siegel, then a research psychopharmacologist at UCLA, proposes a "fourth drive" that is part of animal nature: a motivation for intoxication (207–27). "Like sex, hunger, and thirst, the fourth drive to pursue intoxication can never be repressed. It is biologically inevitable" (210). Referring to a nineteenth century socialite cocaine addict and to Daniel, a young man who had a terrifying experience after drinking datura tea, Siegel expressed this interspecies drive in a particularly lyrical paragraph.

> Annie's dance to the power of this feeling was done in the footsteps and tracks of people and animals who have been inspired by the same beat throughout history. It began with Daniel's *Datura* hop through the woods, along a path strewn with accidental encounters. It was where Kaldi's goats pranced with coffee while livestock staggered on range poisons or galloped in addicting circles for locoweed. There were cats who leaped and turned for catnip while creatures

everywhere twitched, shook, flipped, and rolled to a symphony of hallucinogens. Almost everyone caroused and reeled with alcohol or glided in opium. Mice jumped to the tune of morphine withdrawal. Grasshoppers did it awkwardly with marijuana resin. Llamas stepped assuredly with coca, and rats couldn't stop with cocaine. And primates, great and small, selected a variety of chemical partners, from tobacco to ergot, so they could dance with their ancestors and gods. (210)

Siegel proposes that intoxication may be an odd side effect of beneficial genes that deter us from plants that are truly toxic. Dizziness, sickness, nausea, bad taste, impaired perceptions and movements may be biological warning systems that alert us to the dangers of more deadly poisons. In addition to warning us about real dangers, our warning systems also get activated by less dangerous plants and chemicals and by early weak doses of toxins. Some people, he recognizes, enjoy these changes in perception, especially dizziness. Although Siegel admits that some drugs provide pleasure, he does not recognize possible uses for creative problem solving, creativity, providing a full map of our minds, psychotherapy, producing useful mindbody states, spiritual development, or most of the other fruitful benefits described in this book.

The Most Astonishing, All-time Athletic Feat Ever

There are plenty of other areas of study that intersect with psychedelics, some that engage the human mind, some quirky, some that we will have to omit, but there is a unique, outstanding achievement in athletics that outshines them all.

Perceptual distortions, space warping, time expanding and contracting, awareness of one's body that comes and goes, distracting thoughts, overpowering sounds, shifting colors, almost tangible smells, and powerful emotions are common experiences with psychedelics. How well would a professional athlete perform under such conditions? Not well, we would have to guess, but on June 12, 1970, in San Diego Stadium, in a game between the Pirates and the Padres, pitcher Dock Ellis pitched a no-hitter while on LSD (Hall 1989; Witz 2010). For a delightful four-and-a-half minute cartoon rendition, see: www.dockshort.com/dockshort. I suppose to people who have never done LSD the result is sort of interesting. To people who are experienced, it is astounding, and is, as Jim Fadiman said, "probably the greatest athletic feat of all time, ever."

SUMMARY

These scholarly examples and amusing tastes are not full reviews of psychedelic studies, but they exemplify how varied disciplines are incorporating psychedelics into their studies—or how they might do so if they decide to catch up. These tributaries challenge current scholars and other mischief makers to explore their respective fields from a psychoactive perspective in four ways: 1) search the literature to see what has already been done; 2) psychedelics as a topic of study itself; 3) ask how a current topic of study varies in other mindbody states; and 4) when it becomes legal to do so, work on professional problems and develop insights experimentally the way Harman and his coauthors demonstrated in 1966.

When psychedelics generate attention on previously neglected aspects of human history, culture, and a variety of disciplines, when they provoke questions that scholars and scientists had not asked previously, when they suggest ideas for new methods to study a topic, they might be called *ideagens*.

11

It's a Perinatal World

HITLER AND WAR, SARTRE AND MESCALINE, SNOW WHITE AND FIGHT CLUB

Psychedelics amplify or magnify human psychological experiences. In addition to the contributions we have already touched upon, psychedelics contribute a set of birth-related multistate concepts to the house of intellect, particularly through the work of Stanislav Grof, the world's leading expert on the clinical uses of LSD.* His map of the human mind is a largely untapped reservoir of fertile ideas for insights into our minds, thoughts, emotions, and actions. His theories bring to light new aspects that otherwise would remain hidden and draw our attention to a set of previously unexamined psychological underpinnings.

Using LSD as a sort of microscope for the mind, psychiatrist Grof conducted more than 4,000 sessions, sometimes individually, sometimes as a member of a clinical team. He has also had his own experiences and access to the records of additional sessions. Thus, Grof's sample of the human mind is immense. In *Higher Wisdom,* psychiatrists Roger Walsh and Charles Grob note, "He has therefore perhaps seen a vaster panoply of human experience than anyone else in history" (2005, 119). Just as the microscope benefited biology and medicine by allowing scientists to

---

*The implications of his findings go far beyond psychotherapy (see http://stanislavgrof .com/grofcv.htm.).

assemble hundreds of individual pictures into detailed pictures of the human body, Grof has pieced together a map of the human mind from thousands of separate close-up views.

His map moves our understanding of our minds forward by integrating aspects of perceptual, Freudian-psychodynamic, Rankian-birth, and Jungian collective unconscious psychologies, as well as Eastern psychologies, into one overall model. We are lucky to have this advanced model to draw on. As shown in figure 11.1, the model has four levels: abstract and aesthetic, psychodynamic, perinatal, and transpersonal. As part of the psychodynamic level, Grof presents the concept of clumps of emotion, physical sensations, memories, and bioenergy, which he refers to as COEX, meaning "systems of condensed experiences." In our minds experiences that share the same emotion such as fear, guilt,

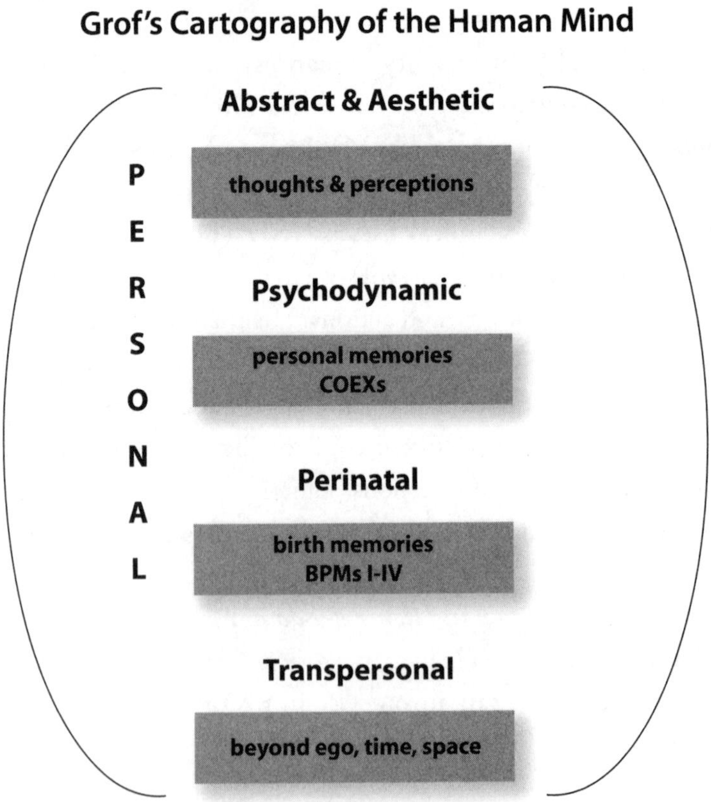

Grof's Cartography of the Human Mind

Abstract & Aesthetic

P
E
R
S
O
N
A
L

thoughts & perceptions

Psychodynamic

personal memories
COEXs

Perinatal

birth memories
BPMs I-IV

Transpersonal

beyond ego, time, space

Figure 11.1. Stanislav Grof's four levels of the mind

abandonment, and so forth clump together; each similar new life experience adds to the accumulation. So, when we experience, say, feeling oppressed—whether socially, physically, or politically—we may react not just to the immediate event but to its whole COEX.

While a COEX's home base is in the autobiographical level, it has deeper origins in the perinatal and transpersonal levels.

> A typical COEX system consists of many layers of unconscious material that share similar emotions or physical sensations; the contributions to a COEX system come from different levels of the psyche. The more superficial and accessible layers contain memories of emotional or physical traumas from infancy, childhood, and later life. On a deeper level, each COEX system is typically connected to a certain aspect of the memory of birth—a specific BPM; the choice of this matrix depends on the nature of the emotional and physical feelings involved. . . . The deepest roots of COEX systems underlying emotional and psychosomatic disorders reach into the transpersonal domain of the psyche. (Grof 2012, 31–32)

THE PERINATAL LEVEL

At first it seems ridiculous that our births can influence us. How can birth be remembered if our brains are not yet developed enough to have thoughts and memories? Much of the antimemory argument centers on the fact that the immature neurons in a newborn's brain do not have their myelin coating, which insulates them from "short-circuiting," so to speak. However, developmental psychologists and medical scientists do recognize that the first hour, or even minutes, of a newborn's life have important psychological effects—bonding—even though the baby's brain is not sufficiently myelinized; contradictorily, then they claim that all the hours of contractions and struggle through the birth canal cannot form a memory because the brain is not sufficiently myelinized. In "Taking Birth Trauma Seriously," Thomas Riedlinger, a master of theological studies from Harvard Divinity School and a fellow of the

Royal Linnaean Society, and pharmacologist June Riedlinger proposed that these memories may be somatic imprints that affect the body and brain via "subcortical learning mechanism" (1986, 20) rather than cognitive-type memories. It is well known that some medical drugs that pregnant women once took had undesirable effects on their fetuses. These, in a sense, were "remembered" biologically, in biological structures. Traumatic events such as birth are also both physical traumas and biochemical ones. Perhaps they are remembered by our bodies too.

The Life Effects of Perinatal Stress

Supporting evidence comes from several directions. The Association for Prenatal and Perinatal Psychology and Health and its journal are developing this field. A study done at Perth's Telethon Institute for Child Health Research in Western Australia asked 2,900 pregnant women about major perinatal stressors such as losing a job, relationship problems, death in the family, financial problems, and similar events then measured their later effects on their children. The well-respected journal *Development and Psychopathology* reported the results (Robinson et al. 2011). When analyzing the information, researchers adjusted for economic and sociodemographic background. The mother's experience of life stress events and child behavioral assessments were also recorded when the children were ages 2, 5, 8, 10, and 14 years.

The results indicate that the number of stressors rather than their kind or their timing are most important. Registered psychologist Dr. Monique Robinson, the lead researcher, said, "Two or fewer stresses during pregnancy are not associated with poor child behavioural development, but as the number of stresses increase to three or more, then the risks of more difficult child behaviour increase" ("Repeated Stress" 2011). The researchers made a point of emphasizing that stressors do not automatically doom a child to bad behavior. The statistical findings applied only to a large number of cases, and, in keeping with Grof's theory, a warm, loving childhood—the personal history level— can help overcome perinatal stress. As Dr. Robinson added, "Regardless of exposure to stress in the womb, once they are born, the right nurturing environment can provide the child with enormous potential to change their course of development. This is known as 'developmental plasticity,' which means that the brain can adapt and change as the child grows with the right environment" ("Repeated Stress" 2011).

Suicide and Birth Experiences

A study of suicide in Sweden highlights the importance of birth experiences. The study compared 242 adults who committed suicide between 1987 and 1995 by violent means such as firearms, jumping from a height, jumping in front of a train, cutting, hanging, or strangulation with 403 siblings born during the same period. Looking for the causes of this difference, Bertil Jacobson of Sweden's Karolinska Hospital and his coauthor Professor Marc Bygdeman found that people who had stressful births were more likely to commit violent suicide than were their brothers or sisters (1998). By no means did all the stressful births result in suicide; this was not the point of the study.

Their results confirmed those of another study, "Perinatal Origin of Adult Self-destructive Behavior," published eleven years previously, which pointed out that the type of suicide was associated with the type of stress at birth, thus, "suicides involving asphyxiation were closely associated with asphyxia at birth, suicides by violent mechanical means were associated with mechanical birth trauma and drug addiction was associated with opiate and/or barbiturate administration to mother during labor" (Jacobson et al. 1987, 364). Whatever the reasons and however unknown the mechanism are, some sort of unconscious memories of birth have a continuing influence.

A Prelude to Drug Use?

An interesting observation about a birth-connected interest in drugs emerges. Statistically, drug administration to the mother, and presumably the fetus, showed up later as a stronger than normal propensity for drug addition. Of course, not always, just a statistical propensity. Is there a perinatal clue here? Transfer from the horrors of being trapped during the contractions of the womb and struggling through the birth canal to emergence with its sense of victory and life is a singular major achievement in independent human existence. If it was accomplished while psychoactive drugs were in the baby's bloodstream, would this unconsciously link drugs with ending the birth trauma and the relief and success of birth? Could this contribute to several generations' fascination with psychoactives as beneficial? If our first, greatest, and life-giving achievement was under drug influence, wouldn't that psychological subbasement provide an unconscious foundation for accepting drug use later in life?

THE FOUR BASIC PERINATAL MATRICES

There are four stages in Grof's perinatal level. Grof calls these clusters Basic Perinatal Memories (BPMs) and sees them as forming an unconscious foundation for our post-birth personalities. Subsequent life experiences attach their feelings (both emotional and physical) to their corresponding BPMs (1975). I find it is handy to think of the BPMs as like four computer folders. Each contains numerous experience-derived files. In addition to the files that come from our birth-related experiences, as we live our lives, our new experiences get saved in the BPM folders, holding similar feelings and emotions.

Good Womb and Bad
BPM I is life in the womb, usually the "good womb," and typically provides feelings of relaxation with all needs being taken care of; however, some fetuses experience a "bad womb" and many fetuses may experience bad episodes.

Contractions
BPM II, the "no-exit hell," starts with contractions, when the cervix is not open enough; typical feelings are those of being trapped with no hope of escape. The late-life entrapments may be physical or emotional, as when one is trapped in a bad relationship or job.

Birth Canal, Titanic Struggle

Grof calls BPM III "titanic struggle." It occurs as we struggle down the birth canal; movies and TV shows often spend most of their time expressing and evoking the feelings of action-based BPM III. They often go back and forth between BPM III and II as heroes and heroines fight, are successful, are trapped again . . . and so on.

Emergence, Success

Finally, BPM IV happens when the baby emerges; it is accompanied by feelings of success, glory, celebration, and triumph. Grof's BPM series provides an exceedingly fertile collection of observations and ideas for the social sciences and the arts, as well as for psychiatry.

PERINATAL ANALYSIS

We use our minds in everything we do, so when a new model of our minds appears, it provides a new way to understand our thoughts and actions. The possibilities are endless; now we will look at some perinatal aspects of politics and the rhetoric of war, mescaline's influence on existentialism, and the movies *Snow White* and *Fight Club*. This is not to say that perinatal analysis is a full analysis. Clearly it is not. But it adds an otherwise missing psychological depth to our understanding, and without it, our analyses are incomplete.

We Are Susceptible to War Rhetoric—
Perinatal Politics and History, Hitler and War

An altogether original insight into history and politics comes from Grof's map of the human mind. The map as a whole and especially the perinatal level provide fertile sets of ideas for analyzing human events. He traces one root of humanity's bellicosity to a deep, unresolved memory of our own birth experiences. Every psychology provides its own psychohistory and psychology of war, and Grof points to unresolved birth struggle as a major root.

In "Perinatal Roots of Wars, Totalitarianism, and Revolutions,"

Grof presents an insightful model for political analysis that deserves elaboration. For example, Hitler's rhetoric was filled with birth imagery that may betray aspects of his own unconscious and may have struck a resonant chord of similar hidden layers in the German people in the 1930s. "A leader such as Hitler is perhaps more strongly influenced by perinatal energies than others in his culture while at the same time having the power to manipulate the collective behavior of an entire nation" (1977, 216). How did some of these perinatal images and themes appear?

BPM I, the good womb—a perfect womb as an imagined past golden age of the Aryan people; a nurturing Motherland

BPM II, no-exit hell—the economic and geographical contractions from losing WWI (war reparations, threatening enemies, lost land); Germany feeling trapped, helpless, victimized, and strangled, paralleling the start of birth contractions before the cervix is open, giving rise to a desire for expansion, *Lebensraum* (room to live in)

BPM III, cosmic struggle—the solution to feeling trapped is cosmic struggle of mythic proportions, war; Hitler imagining himself guiding his folk through the great effort of the birth canal to finally emerge into

BPM IV, a new life—Valhalla, glorious victory and the birth of the thousand-year Reich

Charting the symbolic imagery and psychological aspects preceding wars and revolutions, psychohistorian Lloyd de Mause examined how military leaders can successfully mobilize masses of peaceful civilians and transform them into killing machines. Drawing on Grof, he tracked seventeen instances from Alexander the Great through Napoleon, Hitler, Khrushchev, and Kennedy. As Grof reports, "He was struck by the extraordinary abundance of figures of speech, metaphors, and images related to biological birth that he found in this historical material" (Grof 1977, 214).

Both as individual people and as nations and groups, we are vulnerable to perinatal words, symbolism, imagery, and rhetoric. When people feel trapped as in BPM II, the way out is the aggression of BPM III. These give us a short "war fuse" that is easy to ignite. But recognizing this may dampen the fuse and clear out the deep, dangerous, unconscious memories of our births; perinatal psychotherapy may inactivate these emotional explosives. At the very least, even without therapy we can resist these images once we recognize them. Political columnists, analysts, and commentators would fill their professional roles better if they would alert the public to politicians who use dangerous symbolic birth imagery and perinatal vocabulary that promotes scapegoating or pulls us toward international war and other intergroup conflict. The diplomatic corps and intelligence agencies should have their antennas tuned in for birth imagery too.

When my Psychedelic Studies class meets in the fall of election years, students use perinatal analysis to gain insights into election rhetoric. Sometimes candidates do not use perinatal vocabulary but stimulate the feelings of BPM folders with symbols or putative "dangerous" situations. The threatening enemy may not be a foreign country, but another political party.

Perinatal Philosophy—Sartre and Mescaline

Along a more scholarly vein, Thomas Riedlinger's analysis of Jean Paul Sartre's mescaline experience demonstrates how to use Grofian analysis to discover some of philosophy's psychological roots. Riedlinger, editor of *The Sacred Mushroom Seeker: Essays for R. Gordon Wasson,* has written on religious history and the entheogenic uses of psychedelics.

While Sartre's mescaline experience is not unknown among his readers, it is often dismissed as an odd and meaningless bit of autobiographical trivia, but perinatal theory draws our attention to the experience and shows how it may have influenced his thought and contributed to his fame. After Sartre's mescaline experience, when Simone de Beauvoir, Sartre's longtime companion, telephoned Sartre, he seemed to be in what we would recognize as the feelings and thoughts of being trapped in the no-exit hell of BPM II or cosmic struggle of BPM III. "He said that the phone call had rescued him from a desperate battle with an octopus"—a constricting, crushing BPM II foe. Other threatening hallucinations were umbrellas that turned in to vultures, shoes that became skeletons, and faces that looked monstrous. "Giant beetles and an orangutan's leering face appeared at the window" (Riedlinger 1982, 105). At that time he was twenty-nine years old, an unknown college philosophy teacher, unpublished.

When resolved, the psychological effects of mescaline usually last only several hours, but Sartre's lasted several months, remaining unresolved, so there must have been some nondrug source of them too. Were they tapping in to his unconscious childhood or birth memories? "Sartre insisted that the drug was not primarily responsible. He termed its effect 'incidental,' as compared to the 'profound' cause: A pervasive identity crisis of moving from his passage to adulthood" (Riedlinger 1982, 106).

In addition to tracing Sartre's negative experiences to an unresolved emotional cluster of negative life experiences (a negative COEX on the psychodynamic level in Grof's terms), Riedlinger traces themes in Sartre's philosophy and social commentary to the way the mescaline experience uncovered and amplified Sartre's life experiences, bringing them into his consciousness, and thus coloring his worldview and his writings, particularly the sense of existential crisis, and a typical BPM II thought of meaninglessness. In addition, the mescaline experience seems to have put Sartre in touch with the senseless and interminable suffering of BPM II.

Why would a meaningless existentialism especially appeal so much to France at that time? Why would the sense of being helplessly crushed by powerful forces catch the spirit of the times? In less than a century France had been defeated by Germany, first in the Franco-Prussian War, then World Wars I and II, with a financial depression thrown in for good measure. One would certainly feel a victim of the senseless great tides of history and try to construct a life of meaning for oneself.

Perinatal Cinecrit

Grof's perinatal stages help make sense of many movies and TV shows too. BPM IIIs especially provide rich material for movies. I suppose one reason is that most of us have BPM III in our minds and like to see these inner BPMs acted out. Additionally, I think many people like adrenaline rushes, and BPM III-based violent scenes pump the juice.

Snow White

In Disney's *Snow White and the Seven Dwarfs* the sequence of Snow White's flight-through-the-woods is an especially powerful perinatal sequence. At this point in the movie the queen has instructed the huntsman to take Snow White into the woods and kill her, bringing her heart back in a box. At the beginning of the sequence Snow White is picking flowers in a sunny wooded glade, a beautiful BPM I (primal union with mother) scene. Although we know that the huntsman has brought her here to cut out her heart, she does not know it yet and enjoys the singing birds and flowers of a sunny sylvan day without a care in the world.

After placing a fledging back in its nest (she is a fledgling out of her nest too, but she does not know it), the BPM II experience of being trapped with no escape comes as she is stuck between a rock and a hard place. Literally, she has her back up against a huge boulder as the huntsman, knife in hand, bears down on her.

A splendid BPM III (titanic struggle) sequence begins. The early Disney cartooning is especially good at BPM III. She rushes from the sunny glade into dark and threatening woods. During her symbolic struggle through the birth canal, the trees take on monstrous forms, grabbing at her. Evil glowing eyes follow her and become increasingly malevolent. She falls into an underground river filled with gaping-jawed alligators. She gives up hope, and the screen goes dark.

According to Grof, in the death-rebirth struggle from BPM III to BPM IV (birth, success, victory), "The agonizing experiences culminate, the propulsion through the birth canal is coming to the end, and finally the ultimate intensification of tension and suffering is followed by sudden relief and relaxation" (Grof 1975, 138).

Snow White awakens to a BPM IV forest with cute animals, flowers, birds. She has been psychologically reborn. From there she crosses a stream and enters "transpersonal-land" where the seven dwarfs dwell. There she exhibits the energetic activity to improve the world that typifies BPM IV for some people: "Whistle While You Work."

This summary does not do justice to either Grof's perinatal level or Disney's movie, but it does illustrate how perinatal ideas can help us understand why some works of art have lasting appeal: we were all born, and theoretically we all have these memories stored deep in our minds, ready to be activated by works of art and life experiences. Caesarian births give a different emphasis to BPMs depending on whether they are emergency or elective, but it is beyond the scope of this book to discuss them.

Fight Club

On the surface, *Snow White* and *Fight Club* could hardly be more different. They differ in place, time, characters, tone, plot, and more than six decades of cinema technology, but the same perinatal themes appear (Kackar and Roberts 2005). Both plots portray their main characters' inner battles, which are told—as esteemed mythologist Joseph Campbell says—as if they were happening outwardly in the world. *Snow White* tracked a pubescent heroine as she struggled with her growth toward maturity. *Fight Club* tracks an unnamed male narrator (N), probably in his twenties, who misidentifies with an inner self named Tyler Durden and who battles against this inner false self. Sometimes Tyler, and sometimes N, is in charge.

At the outset N finds himself in a meaningless BPM II. His life is a world of a boring job, a lonely existence, accumulating the "right" furniture and apartment trappings. When he sees everything in his apartment tagged with its price tag, he sees himself caught up in a consumption rat race. When he thinks that corporations will buy naming rights to stars, galaxies, and planets, much as they have bought naming rights to sports venues, he sees himself caught up in the corporate treadmill rat race. N and his inner Tyler are trapped in a BPM II world. Grof expresses some feelings on the part of our minds as "meaninglessness and absurdity of human existence; 'cardboard world,' or the atmosphere of artificiality and gadgets" (1975, 105).

Another BPM II characteristic is a feeling of going insane. Due to insomnia, N develops a blurred or distorted vision of reality and is confused about whether certain events are happening for real or only in his imagination. "With insomnia," he says, "nothing is real. Everything is far away. Everything is a copy of a copy of a copy." As Grof says of BPM II, "subjects feel that they have lost all mental control and become permanently psychotic" (121).

The escape from BPM II, of course, is BPM III. Tyler takes over, and N (controlled by Tyler) acts out the cosmic struggle of BPMs by joining fight clubs, whose members' activity is beating each other. His fascination with the death-rebirth struggle also manifests itself when he joins support groups for people who have fatal diseases. Hayal Kackar, then a doctoral student at Northern Illinois University and the main author of our article on *Fight Club,* identified a rich array of N's additional attitudes and actions that are symptoms of being dominated by BPM III. These include Tyler's Hitler-like behavior as leader of the club. Tyler's imagery and leadership seem to echo Hitler's: they both express BPM III elements.

In spite of a car crash that could have been a BPM IV resolution for N, Tyler is still there. N puts a gun (symbolic?) to his mouth and pulls the trigger. Tyler dies, and N has a rebirth as someone who has integrated and overcome his Tylerness, his BPM III-ness. Finally in charge of his own life, he tells Marla, his girlfriend, "Trust me. Everything's going to be fine."

Again, I am not saying that Grofian psychocriticism presents a complete understanding of *Fight Club* or any other work of art. But our minds produce art, and Grof provides a mind map that informs us of one way our minds go about their work.

Brainstorm

Aware artists intuitively feel what works as they create the images, words, or sounds to fit their creation. In 1937 Disney couldn't have used Grof's map of the mind, which wasn't published until 1975, but in 1983 Douglas Trumbull intentionally used it in the making of *Brainstorm,* in which a death sequence was modeled after Grof's perinatal stages.

Why would a death scene use BPM imagery? In *Beyond Death,* their 1980 study of how death has been portrayed over the centuries and across cultures, the Grofs report strong links between death and how it is portrayed often as rebirth. Death is portrayed as consistent with the BPMs and especially strongly with the death-rebirth transition from BPM III to BPM IV. Calling on their knowledge of how birth is pictured, Trumbull asked the Grofs to help out; in the movie's credits they are listed as consultants for the experiential sequences. It is easy to miss the brief BPM III imagery, but worth watching for. For what it is worth, Hollywood publicity agents claimed that some people became so uncomfortable with the brief special effects of the death scene—read "birth canal scene"—that they left the theater. I expect that in the long run *Brainstorm* will be noted as the first movie to construct its special effects around Grof's theory.

Birth experiences lie deep in our minds where the perinatal level forms a sub-basement under our autobiographical basement. Just as our habitual ways of feeling, thinking, and acting influence our daily lives, they also ignite these perinatal sources and their corresponding emotions. The BPMs flow (sometimes erupt) into our minds. Works of art can powerfully resonate with COEXs in our psychodynamic level and activate BPMs on the perinatal level too.

FOUR-LEVEL GROFIAN ANALYSIS

The other three levels of Grof's theory can apply to movies too. In applying the four-level theory to movies, literature, and other expressions of art, it is helpful to remember that the greatest artistic expression lasts across ages and extends across cultures. Why? What is its widespread appeal? One reason—and there may be others too—is that major works of art, religions, legends, and myths "ring true" because our unconscious minds resonate with them. In *The Hero with a Thousand Faces*, mythologist Joseph Campbell expressed it this way, "The passage of the mythological hero may be over-ground, incidentally; fundamentally it is inward—into depths where obscure resistances are overcome, and long lost, forgotten powers are revivified, to be made available for the transfiguration of the world" (1968, 29). This psychological archaeology is also what goes on when psychedelics are used in psycholytic psychotherapy—using small doses to explore the deeper parts of our minds. Working from quite different directions, from mythology for Campbell and from psychotherapy for Grof, they separately discovered similar mental structures. Here is another lead for cognitive studies, one that includes the humanities.

This intersection showed up when Campbell read a manuscript of what would become Grof's *Realms of the Human Unconscious*. He wrote, "And I have found so much of my thinking about mythic forms freshly illuminated by the findings reported, that I am going to try in these last pages to render a suggestion of the types and depths of consciousness that Dr. Grof has fathomed in his searching of our inward sea" (Campbell 1982, 21). Whether plumbed inwardly with psychotherapy or expressed outwardly in myths and symbols, our inner unconscious sea is sometimes also conveyed in movies, and Grof's four-level map of our minds helps us see this, demonstrated here by *Snow White* and *Pink Floyd, the Wall*.

Snow White

Grof's first level, the abstract and aesthetic, basically sets the time, place, and some characters. We discover Snow White washing the castle steps and the prince riding up on his horse. She first sees his reflection down a well and runs into the castle afraid but interested enough to coyly look out from behind a curtain.

The psychodynamic or personal history level occurs when the queen is jealous that the prince is paying attention to Snow White. After all, the queen wants to be "the most beautiful one of all." This expresses the mutual envy between youth and maturity. Youth envies older people because they are rich and powerful, while the older person resents youth's beauty, attractiveness, and energy. Of course the queen handles this by telling the huntsman to bring her Snow White's heart in a box, and we move to the perinatal level as we saw above.

After her perinatal adventures in the forest, Snow White enters the transpersonal level when she crosses a bridge over a little stream. The rest of the movie is about her transpersonal adventures, which include meeting the dwarfs (perhaps they are her chakras), communicating with animals (possibly her intuition and parapsychological abilities), and twice going into deeper levels of consciousness (once sleeping in the dwarfs' empty beds and still deeper in the sleeping death brought about by a poisoned apple). During many of the transpersonal scenes mushrooms appear. Finally she unites with the prince and they ride off into the golden castle—of transcendence?—in the sky. I have elaborated on this in chapters 2 and 3 of *Psychedelic Horizons* (2006).

Pink Floyd: The Wall

It is tempting to look for the four-stage sequence of the perinatal level and the four levels of Grof's overall map only as they appear in theoretical sequence; however, in our daily lives and in the movies, they often appear scrambled. In long action films, it is not unusual for the hero or heroine to fight out of a BPM II situation and into BPM III, only to be thrown back into BPM II again in a series of cycles. Rather than strictly sticking to the perinatal sequence, *Pink Floyd: The Wall* portrays clear shifts between Grof's levels of our minds. Again, this is not the intent of the movie makers but happens because as aware artists they are in touch with their own minds. They feel what "works."

The movie presents a day in the life of a bum-tripping musician, "Pink," who rockets around his mind's levels. As the camera zooms in to his eye, the opening lyrics clearly state, "If you wanna find out what's behind these cold eyes / You'll have to claw your way through this disguise." This lyric lets us know we are embarking on a psychological adventure into Pink's mind.

The disguised persona that Pink presents to the world is one of his "walls." Emotional themes of abandonment, anger, rage, guilt, fear, loneliness, and loss on his personal history level plunge him into the same themes at deeper and more severe perinatal and transpersonal levels. This illustrates one of Grof's points: the events in our lives may connect to our minds at several levels simultaneously, not just one. Psychodynamic events of the second level may have roots in the third, perinatal level, which may connect with the fourth level's transpersonal imagery and feelings.

In effect, we're seeing the hero Pink dive down from the reality of the abstract and aesthetic level and ricochet among autobiographical memories and fantasies of his personal history, perinatal, and transpersonal levels. Powerful animation marks his perinatal BPMs and occasionally plumbs into the ego-warping, time-warping, and space-warping of his transpersonal unconscious.

The scenes of the abstract and aesthetic level largely take part in a trashed hotel room where he is absorbed with drugs and drug paraphernalia and later in the film at a garishly violent concert where his band is playing; both are seen through his drugged mind. From time to time, these give way to boyhood COEX memories, done in a visual style reminiscent of old photographs. In powerful animation we see Pink sinking to the lower levels. "Behind these cold eyes" the images and memories take on perinatal and transpersonal flavors as mythopoetic themes and archetypal images dominate. Like many movies, BPM III forms the themes of most of the action scenes, and in *Pink Floyd* the major themes of this stage all appear: titanic struggle, aggressive and sadomasochistic, sexual, demonic, scatological, and fiery.

In the "trial scene" in the last few minutes of *Pink Floyd,* psychologically extreme animation adrenalizes its viewers, elaborates earlier themes, and mixes them with magnified, psychedelicized intensity. If there were an award for adult animation (as opposed to kiddie pics), I would certainly nominate these last scenes of *Pink Floyd: The Wall.* In a cataclysmic cathartic finale, Pink breaks down his psychological wall. By knocking down the wall of cold, emotional separateness that led him to live a meaningless life as a brick in society's many walls, Pink expresses and then expels his anger, rage, loneliness, and other interior psychological demons.

The movie ends with a short BPM IV scene. With light, uplifting music, we see young children cleaning up after what looks like both the rubble from a WW II bombing raid and debris from a post-concert riot. One boy picks up a Molotov cocktail, unplugs its rag-fuse stopper, and pours out the gasoline. Another picks up bricks and places them in a new plastic toy truck. Others help clean up the mess. Presumably, Pink can now clean up his life mess.

THE MIND EXPLORER AS HERO

In exploring the frontiers of science fiction, movies have seen an evolution from space adventures and electronic technologies to mindbody adventures that parallel the psychotechnologies of their times. Calling on the technologies of the Victorian era, early movies relied on their clunky, now quaint, contemporary technologies, such as in Jules Verne's spaceship and submarine and the time-traveling chair in *The Time Machine.*

Perinatal movie interpretation and LSD psychotherapy alert us to another kind of hero's journey, that of the mindbody explorer. Grof expressed this theme in a psychotherapeutic context, "As the psychedelic process continues and the subjects explore the world of transpersonal phenomena . . . [t]he universe ceases to be a gigantic assembly of material objects; it becomes an infinite system of adventures in consciousness" (1980, 230). The consciousness hero or heroine faces inner demons and fears of nightmarish intensity, battles them in their outward world reality, and usually overcomes them.

Drugs were portrayed as evil destroyers in older movies such as *Dr. Jekyll, The Man with the Golden Arm,* and the dungeon scene from *Snow White* where the queen drinks the evil brew to transform into the murderous peddler. Now psychotechnology films treat drugs as invitations to the mind-as-frontier, sometimes frightening, sometimes beneficial, often both. *Avatar* and *The Matrix* are transition films:

drugs are mindbody adjuncts that prepare their heroes to plug information directly into their nervous systems—a digitally wired chair in *The Matrix* and plug-together tails in the advanced Navi. *Altered States, Brainstorm,* and *Pink Floyd: The Wall* are early mindbody films. Among the newer members of this genre are *Inception* and *Limitless:* in these twenty-first-century movies, psychoactive drugs produce beneficial extensions of human abilities. Does this mark a cultural shift toward the mindbody explorer as hero?

SUMMARY

The world of ideas flourishes when ideas in one field inform those from others. Psychedelic studies provide new concepts to think with and to hybridize with existing ideas. For example, in this chapter we have glimpsed some examples that occur when perinatal theory intersects with some parts of the rhetoric of war and politics, philosophy, and film criticism. Grof's map of our minds alerts researchers to innovative roads in their specialties, framing new research agendas and questions. Most important, the human mind is the universal tool that all sciences, humanities, arts, and applied fields use. By giving us a more detailed view of our mind's strengths and weaknesses, Grof's theory upgrades our skill in using this all-inclusive tool.

12

The Neurosingularity Project

WHEN BIGGER HEADS AND BETTER BRAINS SURPASS OUR CURRENT ONES

Psychedelics—whether used for psychotherapy or personal growth—contribute to a much larger project, which I call the "Neurosingularity Project." As the name immediately suggests, it derives from Ray Kurzweil's adaptation of the scientific word *singularity*, to refer to a hypothetical future emergence of greater-than-human superintelligence through technological means for the title of his 2005 book, *The Singularity Is Near: When Humans Transcend Biology*. He proposes a time not long from now when computers will think more skillfully than humans, thanks to nanotechnology, genetics, and artificial intelligence. But as the subtitle suggests, Kurzweil assumes that human brains and their biological information processing are static while computers and electronic information processing surpass our poor outdated brains.

Neurosingularity is a rough parallel and posits a time when future human brains (and minds) will function significantly better than our brains today. We have two parallel and mutually supporting singularities, electronic and biological. Rather than just speeding up information processing, neurosingularity is likely to increase the variety of biology-based information processing. Can we build better brains and install a greater variety of biological information processing programs, that is, more mindbody states?

According to multistate theory, there are vast and unknown numbers of mindbody states, each with its own kinds of cognitive and noncognitive functioning. We achieve/install these states by using a variety of psychotechnologies. Although this book focuses only on the psychedelic family, a complete Neurosingularlity Project would explore all known techniques for moving toward superior brains and eagerly await other psychotechnologies yet to be discovered or invented. In this context the word *brains,* of course, is too restricting, but it will serve as a shorthand for our whole nervous system and hormonal system, as well as other aspects of our bodies.

Unfortunately most people who are investigating the wide range of psychotechnologies do not see their own work or that of others as integrated into a larger picture. However, the ideas of multistate theory and Neurosingularity Project will aid recognition that all mindbody tributaries flow into a much grander river.

The rivers that flow into the Neurosingularlity Project vary from millennia-old plant-based shamanism (Schultes and Hofmann 1992), through today's neurosciences and traditional breeding-based genetics, to emerging specialties such as medical genetics and transgenics (in which DNA from a different species is inserted into an organism). As this chapter speculates, future developments may result in both more efficient current brains and newly designed ones with new neurotransmitters, new receptor sites, and other new structures. In this chapter we'll look at some leads, extend them into the future, and speculate on what may develop. Compared with earlier chapters, this one is more high-flying and speculative, so take it with a grain of salt—or whatever you like to flavor your mind with.

NEUROSCIENCE LEADS

Biology and neuromedicine are generating increasingly detailed descriptions of our nervous system and how it functions. As with other scientific advances, every discovery leads to applications. From pharmacology we will consider drugs used singly and in combinations. From genetics we will look at transgenics and intelligence amplification. In a more speculative vein, we will ask, "Are brain design and synthetic mindbody states in our future?" The following items might best be seen as a list of leads. Some may pan out. Many won't.

Pharmacology

Currently pharmacology is the river with the greatest flow of new psychotechnologies. Its tributary of psychedelics is just one of many contributing to its gigantic flow. Appropriately enough, the synaptic gap between nerve cells is a major focus of pharmacological attention. Some chemicals speed up or increase the amount of neurotransmitters that the sending cells squirt into the gap. Others slow down or decrease the amount. Still others slow down or speed up the scavengers that pick up neurochemicals and recycle them for reuse. On the receiving side of the gap, another group of medicines affect how neurotransmitters plug in to the receiving cells or how the receiving cells react. The discoveries of how our synapses work and other discoveries about our nervous systems are great advances in biology and medicine, and humanity is better off thanks to them. Using modern genetics, it may well be possible to improve their design or even invent new kinds.

As we have seen, historically and culturally most psychedelic use was, and still is, of one plant at a time. In just one publication of a large collection of evidence for the historical and prehistorical use of psychedelic plants, stretching "well back into the Pleistocene"—"Archeological Evidence for the Tradition of Psychoactive Plant Use in the Old World"—more than 180 studies are cited (Merlin 2003, 295). In the past decade there may have been as many more. In the late twentieth century and early twenty-first century, pharmacology has moved beyond naturally occurring substances to scientifically designed molecules.

We are rapidly advancing in our ability to use psychedelics and other psychoactive substances to influence the synaptic sending and receiving cells and their scavengers. An opportunity for growth in one-at-a-time psychotechnology is inventing new psychotechnologies, chemicals, breathing skills, exercise routines, and so forth.

The next step, then, is to combine psychotechnologies into new recipes or to sequence them in innovative series. An early example is found in the suggestion to use two psychoactive drugs to structure psychedelic sessions made by a true pioneer in psychedelics, Myron J. Stolaroff. Stolaroff was vice president for long-range planning at Ampex Corporation, one of the grandparents of Silicon Valley, where magnetic sound recording tape and videotape were developed.

Stolaroff left Ampex to found the International Foundation for Advanced Study (IFAS) in Menlo Park, California. IFAS provided many of the first studies of the use of psychedelics for creativity and problem solving. One of his coworkers there was James Fadiman. Stolaroff also knew many of the other psychedelic pioneers, including the previously elusive "Secret Chief," an underground psychedelic psychotherapist, now identified as psychiatrist Leo Zeff (Stolaroff 2004). Drawing on his years of experience, friendship with psychedelic practitioners, and analysis of how to structure psychedelic sessions, in his book *Thanatos to Eros,* Stolaroff proposes using MDMA first to see if a person is comfortable with altered mindbody experiences, and if so, starting a later session with MDMA to establish a positive emotional set prior to a second stage provided by LSD. Referring to his IFAS period, he reports, "The combination of MDMA followed by LSD proved an extremely effective one" (1994, 54–56).

This instance of combining mindbody psychotechnologies is somewhat odd because it uses two drugs. The combination of meditation and psychedelics has been used far more often. In *Psychedelic Reflections* psychiatrist Roger Walsh gives a sequencing example when he reports that several spiritual leaders whom he interviewed found psychedelic sessions benefited from a prior "period of quiet and/or meditation" (1983, 117). According to the 1996 article "Buddhism and Psychedelics" in the Buddhist journal *Tricycle,* psychedelic experiences piqued many practioners' interest in spiritual matters, leading them away from drugs toward meditation and experiential religions.

GENETIC LEADS

The confluence of genetics and the other rivers of scientific information hasn't happened yet in multistate studies, but when we look at the path that scientific innovation usually takes, it's just a matter of time before it does. The sending cell of a synapse, its neurotransmitters, the receiving cell, and its internal cascade of relayed messages are all made according their respective genetic blueprints. So the next step is to control neuronal cell construction by turning the appropriate genes on and off. As "Functioning Synapse Created Using Carbon Nanotubes" hints, this opens the door to correspondingly more basic levels of medical intervention/treatment, possibly eventually combining with deeper levels of invention via genetics (University of Southern California 2011).

SYNTHETIC BIOLOGY— TRANSGENIC INVENTION

Just as chemists have synthesized new compounds and materials, geneticists are combining biological building blocks, including genes, in new ways, called appropriately "synthetic biology" (*Discover Magazine* 2009). Besides the interventions related to repairing organs and even growing replacements, they are inventing variants of existing plants and animals. A 2011 article "Harvard Scientists to Make LSD Factory from Microbes" describes how biologists have worked with yeast to adapt it to make lysergic acid, a precursor to LSD. This process is the first of several steps in producing LSD and the full sequence is not complete yet, but this advance could be a first step to complete LSD production. Using these techniques, will new psychoactive chemicals and plants be invented?

Genetic engineering also hints at processes that may one day reshape our brains and minds. For example, using gene transfer from one species to another, scientists have introduced a gene for scorpion poison into cabbage, one that is harmless to humans but kills cabbage worms. They have engineered the digestive processes of a pig so that its feces will contain less phytate to cut down on algae blooms when the sewage gets into water, and they have developed chickens whose eggs contain cancer-fighting medicines ("Designer Hens" 2007). More recreationally, by introducing a gene for a green fluorescent protein (GFP) from a jellyfish into a rabbit (Philipkoski 2002) and into a cat ("Glowing Cats" 2011), they have produced animals that glow in the dark under fluorescent light. The GFP is now in labs worldwide where it is used in numerous plants and animals, including flatworms, algae, *E. coli,* and pigs. Glow in the dark marijuana?

Does genetic transfer point to an opening for transgenic scientists who have an interest in psychedelics? Might they transfer genetic material from psilocybin mushrooms into, say, blue cheese mold? Similar opportunities for transfer may exist for genes from marijuana or ergot and other psychoactive plants. The possibilities are exciting.

AMPLIFYING INTELLIGENCE

To a large degree, most discussions of amplifying intelligence are restricted to increases via artificial intelligence (Englebart 1962). However, as we saw in the chapter on enhancing cognition and intelligence, a full consideration of amplifying intelligence has to include pharmacological and biological advances too. The genetic view might be considered science fiction—for the time being at least—until the science catches up with these speculations and applied technologies catch up with the science. Instead of using only electronic information technology—or biology hybridized with IT—to augment human intelligence, advances in genetics are moving us down the path toward producing better human brains.

FROM INSIGHT TO INTERVENTION
TO INVENTION

Is it indeed possible to improve our brains, their structure, and functions? When we look at the road that science and its applications take, they start with discoveries, then move to overcoming current problems, then extend these advances to complex interactions with other applications and then move beyond to inventing things that have not existed yet. If pharmacology and genetics follow the typical three "I's" of science-based progress—insight, intervention, and invention—where might they take us as the years roll by?

Insight

In scientific fields basic discoveries typically occur first. But by no means does this always happen. Skilled craftsmen blended metals when they were still thinking about the spirit of iron and the soul of copper. Some shamans make similar claims about plants. But in our age and culture, scientific insight generally starts the ball rolling.

With new genetic instrumentation, techniques, and discoveries coming on fast, the previously slow-moving rivulet of genetic research is now a rushing torrent. Mapping the human genome,* the functions of its genes, cellular genetics, and the onrush of other discoveries are advancing both science and its technology.

Intervention

Following scientific genetic discoveries, we are seeing the applied stage of the journey. Clinical genetics is a specialty of clinical medicine with particular attention to hereditary disorders, including birth defects, developmental problems, autism, epilepsy, short stature, and many others.

A bioengineering example of insight leading to intervention (and thence to invention) comes from nanotechnology. At the University of Southern California engineering professors built a synthetic synapse, which functions similarly to a brain synapse. The development of nano-tubes and ways to manipulate them was the previous insight step. The team leader, Professor Alice Parker, looks forward to the intervention

---

*There is a somewhat credible report that Watson and Crick, who came up with the double helix model, may have had their insight while on LSD (Rees 2004). But in spite of my hope that it would be nice if it were true, in my judgment it's likely but not proven. However, some people do credit LSD with this insight (Fadiman 2011). I hope they know more about it than I do.

stage, expecting the technology might provide prosthetic devices for brain injury. Her team is already thinking about the invention stage. "The next step is even more complex. How can we build structures out of these circuits that mimic the function of the brain, which has 100 billion neurons and 10,000 synapses per neuron?" Next, she says, is building brain plasticity in the circuits, but a whole synthetic brain or even a brain area is decades away ("Functioning Synapse" 2011). In an increasingly multidisciplinary world, maybe we are seeing the birth of a new field: neuronano engineering. On a more wildly science-fiction note, will it become possible to design genes that build nanostructures or nanofactories that produce genes or proteins? Because they work with similar-size objects, somehow or other, these fields seem destined to hybridize.

Invention: Designing New Neurostructures and Neurotransmitters

Geneticists are now identifying genetic errors that result in dysfunctional diseases (insight), and will soon increase interventions, perhaps by activating genes to help produce more (or less) of a neurotransmitter. Addressing problems regarding the structure of some of the cells that form a synapse is likely to be next. These cells may need more vesicles to squirt out their neurotransmitters or more (or fewer) receptor sites on the receiving cells. While not easy tasks, the possibility of adjusting current processes to accomplish them fits within the usual road of progress in the medical sciences. Perhaps a genetic solution to producing more nerve growth factors will be needed to help overcome a disease or injury. Perhaps chemicals that can activate the appropriate genes can be introduced into our—or future generations'—brains.

However, the blood-brain barrier has to be contended with in any attempt to chemically influence neurons in the brain. This filtering device screens out many molecules but lets through those that the brain needs such as water, oxygen, and glucose. For one hundred years medical and biological researchers have been stumped by the problem of getting chemicals, especially large ones, into the brain. However, researchers at

Cornell University have discovered a molecular key—adenosine—to open the blood-brain doors (Carman et al. 2011). Treatment, as usual, will take precedent over other uses, and diseases such as Alzheimer's, multiple sclerosis, and brain cancers are first in line. But after that, what? Will adenosine doors open the way to nurturing neurons, building better brains, and carrying new psychoactive molecules?

Working along a different line, researchers at Columbia University's departments of bioengineering and radiology have developed another way to open the blood-brain barrier using ultrasound, as documented in "Noninvasive and Localized Neuronal Delivery Using Short Ultrasound Pulses and Microbubbles" (Choi et al. 2011). Until recently the use of relatively strong ultrasound has often caused collateral damage. The new treatment uses much smaller and shorter bursts. After diffusion through the blood-brain barrier, the inserted drugs not only affect cell membranes but can penetrate all the way through to the cell's nucleus. Here too, Alzheimer's is the first target for treatment, but will this method along with the adenosine method also open a door to the brain and innovative psychoactive drugs and new psychotechnologies for delivering them?

On a more science-fiction note: When scientists discover the genes that control nerve growth factors and develop the ability to regulate them, will they be able to assist this natural process in order to produce more brain cells? Will the Neurosingularity Project then move from brain repair and enhancement to enlargement or even brain design? Of course our current skulls are full already, but delaying the hardening of our skulls by a year or more and allowing them to expand even a little would create more room for additional cells.

This is not a prediction, only a speculation, but the speculation is not without some grounding. Craniosynostosis is the premature closing of the skull in babies (affecting about 1 out of 2,500 in the U.S.). Surgeons and engineers at Emory University and the Center for Pediatric Healthcare Technology in Atlanta are developing treatment for craniosynostosis and have developed a model in mice that may be adapted someday to children. In one study they discovered genes that influence fusion in the skull. In another, they designed a gel that can be injected into the gap between skull bones to slow down their premature closing. Currently, of course, their work is for intervention/treatment ("New Hope" 2011). Will it move into an invention stage to promote natural brain growth to continue awhile longer? Something is already naturally happening along these lines. In a study of the brains of Americans, anthropologists at the University of Tennessee at Knoxville reported

> that the average height from the base to the top of the skull in men has increased by eight millimeters (0.3 inch). The skull size has grown by 200 cubic centimeters, a space equivalent to a tennis ball. In women, the corresponding increases are seven millimeters and 180 cubic centimeters. ("Anthropologists Find" 2012)

Big-headed movie creatures from outer space do not seem so odd now. Maybe they're our descendants.

Another clue to this possibility already comes from another genetic discovery. One of the major differences between humans and chimpanzees is that human skulls continue to grow for a longer time than chimp skulls do. According to a study published in *Nature*, "Human-specific Loss of Regulatory DNA and the Evolution of Human-specific Traits," researchers discovered several regulatory genes that turn other genes on and off are active in chimps but turned off in humans (McLean 2011). Gill Bejerano, a researcher at the Howard Hughes Medical Institute and Stanford University School of Medicine, and his colleague, David Kingsley, compared the genetic code of humans to chimpanzees. They looked for genes that existed in chimps but were missing in humans. Even more interesting to Kingsley, however, is that another of the DNA deletions in humans was located near a gene that kept brain cell growth in check. "The deletion of this DNA may have contributed to the development of larger brains in humans," he said (Steenhuysen 2011). In the future, will this lead to a way to build still larger brains? Will it be combined with turning on the genes that control nerve growth factors?

When we look to chemistry and materials engineering and realize what they have accomplished, startling questions emerge. Just as experts in these fields synthesized previously unknown compounds and materials, will neurogeneticists improve on our brains not just by overcoming their current shortcomings with interventions but also by empowering them with additional growth or complexity? Are such things possible? When scientists discover the suites of genes that produce our neurotransmitters, will they be able to turn them on and off?

Will they move beyond that? Will they design new neurotransmatters and new receptor sites to accept them? Will they dare to? When they discover the origins of nerve growth factors, what then? What will happen if scientists activate the genes to produce additional nerve growth factor, which a recent study indicates is possible (Berg et al. 2011)? It's a long way from salamander brains to human brains. Or is it? Perhaps this research will lead to the ability to temporarily control the regulatory genes that control the on/off switch for nerve cell growth. Future generations might not be stuck with the craniums and their contents that we have now.

I am not claiming that researchers are on the verge of transforming our brains and nervous systems, but some of these leads and ones like them may be the grandparents of future psychotechnologies. To keep up on these advances, I recommend a free subscription to *Science Daily*'s "Mind and Brain News" mailing list (www.sciencedaily.com). They also have a news list titled "Illegal Drugs and Controlled Substances News."

ARE WE ALL HIDDEN SAVANTS?

The savant syndrome provides one of many other clues worth following. In April 2011, I attended a bioethics conference in Madison, Wisconsin, sponsored by ProMega Corporation. Dr. Darold A. Treffert, a specialist in savant syndrome from the University of Wisconsin Medical School, described a puzzling case. A surgeon who was struck by lightning via a telephone line just as he was hanging up became a musical savant, while continuing to function normally, including being able to practice surgery (Treffert 2011). This raises the question of whether savant abilities are available to nonsavants if we could develop a psychotechnology to access or install them. A clue comes from Australia.

A whole issue of the *Philosophical Transactions of the Royal Society B: Biological Sciences* was dedicated to the savant syndrome; it included an article by Allan Snyder from the Centre for the Mind in Australia. He proposes that savants "have privileged access to lower level, less-processed information" (Snyder 2009, 1399) in our brains, and in the section "Inducing Savant Skills Artificially" he speculates that "such skills might be artificially induced by low-frequency repetitive transcranial magnetic stimulation" in normal adult brains.

Snyder's whole abstract is exciting reading, not only because it may be a clue to hidden human abilities but also because it illustrates how leads come from strange places.

Abstract. I argue that savant skills are latent in us all. My hypothesis is that savants have privileged access to lower level, less-processed information, before it is packaged into holistic concepts and meaningful labels. Owing to a failure in top-down inhibition, they can tap into information that exists in all of our brains, but is normally beyond conscious awareness. This suggests why savant skills might arise spontaneously in otherwise normal people, and why such skills might be artificially induced by low-frequency repetitive transcranial magnetic stimulation. It also suggests why autistic savants are atypically literal with a tendency to concentrate more on the parts than on the whole and why this offers advantages for particular classes of problem solving, such as those that necessitate breaking cognitive mindsets. A strategy of building from the parts to the whole could form the basis for the so-called autistic genius. Unlike the healthy mind, which has inbuilt expectations of the world (internal order), the autistic mind must simplify the world by adopting strict routines (external order). (1,399)

The abstract meets several criteria of multistate theory. It proposes hidden abilities in our minds, suggests a psychotechnology to access them (transcranial magnetic stimulation), and it fits into the central multistate research question: How do human skills vary in savant mindbody states?

SUMMARY—MIND DESIGN

Without our recognizing it, the Neurosingularity Project has already started down the typical road from scientific insight to intervention/ treatment to invention. Much of the information above marks milestones along this road. Current neuropsychology is mapping the human mind and many of its complexities. There is still a long and exciting way to go. A full map must include all mindbody states and all their respective abilities and biological correlates.

Chapter 8 mentioned the possibility of combining existing mindbody psychotechnologies, both chemical and behavioral, to produce new mindbody states. There we considered only new mindbody states as they might affect our current brains, but genetic sciences raise the possibility not only of enhancing our current brains' activities but also designing advanced brains.

Existing psychotechnologies provide enough leads to keep generations of psychologists, biologists, and their many friends and relations busy. And the scope of the Neurosingularity Project will grow even more as new psychotechnologies are invented and imported from other cultures and the number of mindbody combinations and sequences multiplies. When brain enhancement is added, the number of possible psychotechnology recipes and sequences multiplies again. For future mindbody inventors—perhaps we should we call them *neuroarchitects, neuroengineers, neuroartists,* or *neurodesigners*—the possibilities of the Neurosingularity Project and the human future are endless.

PART 3

From Lab to Life, From Clinic to Campus

In part 1 we looked at the mystical mindbody state and some of the ways it alters other aspects of life. The first chapter of part 2 broadened our perspective and provided a way to look at the wider field of mindbody states. Then chapters 8 through 12 focused on how psychedelics and multistate theory enrich cognitive studies and open new intellectual frontiers.

How can society benefit from these leads? In part 3 we look at three answers. With current research confirming earlier research from the 1960s and 1970s, psychotherapy takes the lead in applications. But findings from clinical research do not magically move from research lab into society. Some sort of institution has to house them. A second problem: in many cases pilot studies are complete, but it takes large-scale, multi-site studies with sophisticated designs to get approval of federal authorities and evidence of effectiveness to receive payments from insurance companies. Such studies are very expensive, often running into the tens of millions of dollars. Chapter 13 proposes one solution to solve both problems, a company whose business is providing professionally guided sessions.

Chapter 14 points out that an enhanced view of the human mind, which includes all mindbody states, naturally expands the meaning of *well educated* to include learning to achieve useful states and to develop their abilities. Additionally, all the questions and topics of current singlestate education get re-asked for education in all other mindbody states. Psychedelics and other psychotechnologies offer vast horizons for universities, research institutions, and foundations.

For universities and colleges, in chapter 15 I present my own Foundations of Psychedelic Studies course as a beginning example of many similar courses that ought to be taught. Having taught this course since 1981, I have developed some useful hints on how to teach psychedelic courses. The course is designed as part of a liberal education for nonspecialists, but most higher education faculties could easily design Psychedelic Studies in (Name of discipline) or Psychedelic (Name of discipline). Thanks to articles in esteemed professional journals such as those mentioned in chapter 1, professors who propose new courses can provide evidence of psychedelics' growing respectability. Parallel courses for other psychotechnologies call for creation too. Medical, legal, religious, and governmental studies and other graduate programs wait to be multistate-enriched too. The opportunities are boundless.

13

Reaching the Unreachable Public While Raising $1+ Billion for Psychedelic R & D via Crowdfunding

A BIZ-FI SPECULATION

The two biggest obstacles to making psychedelics' benefits available to the public are 1) educating the general public—especially influential people—about psychedelics' possible uses and 2) raising funds to finance the costs of research for drug testing and approval. Members of a few organizations are doing some funding, but their number is a minuscule part of the total population. A few informed large donors have provided research funds to get the ball rolling, and they deserve thanks from all humanity for their donations to human welfare. But it will take an enormously larger amount of money to build a database large enough to apply for governmental approvals for the large range of health applications of psychedelics and many millions or even billions more for research on the use of psychedelics for religious, intellectual, artistic, and other purposes, as well as problem solving and cognitive enhancement. One solution can solve both the public knowledge problem and the funding problem at the same time while raising a billion dollars or more: crowdfunding.

A hypothetical dialogue can well present this idea.

VENTURE CROWDFUNDER: A billion dollars? You must be crazy. You'll never get people to donate that much.

TOM ROBERTS: That's right. Large donors have been wonderful in their generosity and thousands of small donors and donor-members to nonprofit organizations like MAPS have supported psychedelic research year after year, but what I have in mind is not donations. To pay for large, multisite, controlled clinical studies, the sources of funds will have to be expanded enormously. The way to do this is via investments.

VC: Right! You mean you're going to manufacture psychedelics and sell them? See you in jail.

TR: No, that's not it. Besides, even if making and selling psychedelics were legal, most people would take them only once or a few times in their lives. They are not like most prescription drugs that people take daily or even several times a day. The money in psychedelics will come from providing sessions—screening clients, preparing them, supporting them during the sessions, and helping them integrate their experiences afterward. Think of the model of dialysis centers or endodontists. It is the professional skills that people pay for.

   The same sort of model can be applied to psychedelics. Partial models for this process are in clinical research settings such as Roland Griffiths's research on meaningfulness and spirituality at Johns Hopkins (Griffiths et al. 2006, 2008) and Michael Mithoefer's (2007, 2011) work with PTSD patients and the studies done by Charlie Grob at UCLA Harbor Hospital (2011) and the Ross-Guss team at NYU Medical School and Bellevue Hospital (2012), which both address overcoming anxiety when facing death.

VC: How would it work?

TR: The professional use of anesthetics is a partial example. People take them only under the direct supervision of a professional anesthesiologist. Similarly people would take psychedelics under the direct supervision of qualified psychedelic professionals (Grof 2001; Johnson et al. 2008). For spiritual uses, qualifications would also have to include being a qualified spiritual guide as described by James Fadiman (2011), Neal Goldsmith (2011), and Robert Jesse (2012). The important thing to notice is that their work represents a professional concern about qualifications as opposed to the psychedelic evangelical enthusiasm of the 1960s. For uses such as creative problem solving and increasing aesthetic sensitivity, the guidelines for guides will have to be worked out, and funding that research and development will be one of the uses of investors' money.

VC: So this would not mean I could get a prescription for LSD, buy it at a drug store, and go home and become music?

TR: Sorry. You'll have to take it with a professional guide on hand, and if you are doing it for a psychotherapeutic reason, you will have to be referred by a mental health professional.

VC: But I want to take it for spiritual development. Does that make me crazy enough?

TR: Sorry again. But the company I imagine—I call it Community Psychedelic Centers International (CPC)—will have two divisions, a psychotherapy division and a personal growth division. CPC's psychotherapy division would offer medical and psychotherapeutic treatments using psychedelics, while the personal development division would offer sessions for uses such as those mentioned above. Both divisions will use both physical and mental screening, preparation, guided sessions, and post-session integration. Maybe you would qualify for the personal growth division. In addition to spiritual growth, that division will provide sessions for creative problem solving, scientific and scholarly insights, artistic inspiration, self-understanding, and similar applications.

VC: Okay. But why would I invest in such a company?

TR: To provide a service that will benefit humanity and at the same time make money. "Doing well by doing good," as the phrase goes. What would the dollar value be for curing post-traumatic stress disorder, alcoholism and addiction, depression, neuroses and psychoses, cluster and migraine headaches, obsessive-compulsive disorder, relationship issues, death anxiety, or autism? This is what would determine the value of CPC's various services. Even if full medical trials show that only a few of these diseases and conditions can be successfully treated, how much would successful treatments and a company that provides them be worth? At this point the leads and pilot studies look promising, but, as with any new venture, there is no promise of success.

VC: Are you kidding? This sounds like a good idea, but more of a pipe dream than a possibility. People are never going to go for it.

TR: Not as things are now. But if society is going to benefit from the apparent multiple potentials of psychedelics, they have to be embedded in acceptable activities within recognized institutions, ones that people know and trust. Psychedelics need to become an "insiders" interest, not just something a few "outsiders" and leftover hippies are toying with. At the present, people who are interested in using psychedelics, even carefully, can be misperceived as being located on the fringes of society. The question is "How do we move psychedelics' benefits from the fringes to the center?" The financial world is certainly one of society's centers, and this is a method of recruiting them. People understand companies that offer services and charge for them. Community Psychedelic Centers International provides two answers—informing the public and raising money to fund research.

Founding a company to provide specialized medical services is something people understand. It fits in with how people know society works, especially how many powerful people think about things. If stockholders are willing to "put their money where their mouth is," the idea gains credibility. A million-dollar company (or a billion-dollar company) that is willing to invest in psychedelic psychotherapy has more credibility than does an isolated research project here or a small, pilot treatment project there.

VC: A multi-million-dollar company or even a billion-dollar company? What have you been smoking?!

TR: The numbers support it; in fact, they oversupport it. According to the *2009 National Survey on Drug Use and Health* 23.6 million Americans have used LSD some time in their lives. Another 14.2 million have used Ecstasy (MDMA): total = 37.8 million. But some people have used both, so let us reduce the Ecstasy number by half to 7.1 million. This gives us a total of 30.7 million. And this doesn't include users of mescaline, peyote, DMT, ayahuasca, and other lesser-known psychedelics (Substance Abuse and Mental Health Services Administration 2010).

Even if we estimate that only 1 percent of this number would invest in CPC, we would get 307,000 investors. If each one invests an average of only $5,000, that gives us a billion and a half dollars plus change. Moreover, this estimate is only past users. That's a small slice of the total U.S. investors' pie. We could also reasonably expect participation from:

- psychedelically naive investors
- "businessman's risk" investors
- venture capitalists
- mutual funds
- banks
- insurance companies
- corporate retirement funds
- pension plans
- sovereign funds
- endowments
- and more

TR: Unlike people who have used psychedelics, most of the people in these groups are not interested in psychedelics per se, much less in states of overwhelming unitive consciousness. They are interested in making money. By appealing to the profit motive, this offering would encourage these groups to become informed about psychedelic research and to invest in a company that offers this cluster of services. Besides this, these groups are a powerful, influential, and dominant part of society.

We have not even considered foreign investors; these may well equal or exceed U.S. investors in their numbers. And wealthy domestic investors may want to invest substantial amounts. I have no idea how many of each of these there are, but a few large investors plus foreign investors would well lift an initial public offering of stock (IPO) to several billion. Invested in research and governmental approval, these funds would speed up treatment for millions of people.

VC: So, if you are starting off with more than $1.5 billion just from psychedelically experienced people in the United States, what is a realistic estimate of how much a company could raise from other investors and worldwide?

TR: I wish I knew. The numbers get very large very fast. I used a $5,000 investment in the example above because it is midrange for most IRA (Individual Retirement Account) yearly investments. These investors might buy stock in their other accounts too. And what if my 1 percent estimate of lifetime users is really 2 percent or 3 percent? Would foreign investors match U.S. investors? How much would venture capitalists, mutual funds, insurance companies, and similar pools of money invest? As much as individuals? More? If even a fraction of these possible sources comes through, several billion dollars is not an unreasonable estimate. If several or all of them invested, those funds would provide a huge amount of support for research on known drug candidates and for discovering and synthesizing new ones, while alleviating suffering for millions of people. Along the way, we'd also learn a great amount about our brains and our minds.

VC: The idea of going public is just too weird.

TR: That is what people thought of a medical marijuana initial public offering in 2001. G. W. Pharmaceutical, Ltd., increased its IPO from what they originally planned. Their IPO doubled the original amount ("G. W. Pharmaceutical" 2001).

Cannabis company GW Pharmaceuticals raises $34.5 mm in IPO

Deal Date: Jun-01-2001 / Deal # 200130273

EXECUTIVE SUMMARY

British biotechnology company GW Pharmaceuticals, which is developing prescription drugs derived from cannabis, raised gross proceeds of $34.5mm (UK25mm) in an oversubscribed initial public offering of almost 13.7mm ordinary shares on the Alternative Investment Market. It had originally expected to raise UK16mm.

VC: IPO? Is that some kind of drug I haven't heard of? What does it do? How do I get some?

TR: IPO means initial public offering of stock; it's when a company first sells its stock to the public. It's a kind of crowdfunding. Unlike donation crowdfunding where control goes to the project head, in investor crowdfunding, you maintain influence over the project and share in its outcome. G. W. Pharmaceutical is Britain's only legal marijuana producer; they are selling a marijuana-derived medicine in Canada, the U.K., continental Europe, and are completing a Phase III study for treating cancer pain in the United States now. Their international marketing partners include Beyer, Novartis, Almirall, and Otsuka. [Disclosure: I own some GWP. —TBR] Can we expect something similar with Community Psychedelic Centers? No one knows, but GWP's history shows that risk-informed investors are out there and willing to invest in possible novel treatments.

VC: Okay, but can CPC make money?

TR: This is *the* question, and we'll know that only after CPC is in business for a couple of years. But there are good reasons to think it can. For now we need a good business plan. We know the evidence so far shows that psychedelics used skillfully as adjuncts to psychotherapy and in safe clinical settings can be effective for several conditions. The exact dollars-and-cents figures and a sound business plan are one of the things CPC's founders will have to develop. In the long run it clearly looks like this service will save money on psychotherapy treatment. Insurance companies and national health plans would benefit.

Wall Street is used to evaluating new technologies, products, services, and processes. It seldom has as much evidence to start with as it does with psychedelics, and it seldom has as much preliminary research already accomplished as it does with CPC. A big task now is building a business model.

VC: Due diligence and fiduciary responsibility are not going to happen overnight.

TR: Yes, but due diligence and fiduciary responsibility are the hidden strengths of this idea. The question "Can CPC make money?" needs to be investigated by brokers, bankers, mutual fund managers, and others in the investment community. To answer it, they will begin to read the research on psychedelics, obtain professional opinions from experts who know the evidence, and generally "ask around." This is part of the process of "due diligence," which entails finding out all the material facts about a corporation before investing.

Due Diligence by Intermediaries
(in general and in this particular case)

Investigation to confirm all material facts about a potential investment

Here: material facts include research on the potential uses of psychedelics

TR: While exercising due diligence for financial and fiduciary reasons, as a side effect, they will learn about psychedelics' history, pilot studies, and ongoing research. Some people in the financial community may become volunteers in certain studies too. As the financial community becomes informed, it and the psychedelic community will join their common interests.

Spreading Information	
It is difficult to get a man to understand something when his salary depends upon his not understanding it.	It is easy to get a man to understand something when his salary (income) depends on his understanding it.
—Upton Sinclair	—Not Upton Sinclair

Additionally, the financial and business communities already have members who are psychedelically informed, so these individuals are already favorably primed. Through the financial and business communities, the wider society will become educated about psychedelics' potentials via this stock offering. This is no mere side effect, no small accomplishment. The IPO is a way to educate the public.

If promising current leads are fulfilled, these treatments will also inform and attract people whose medical conditions might be treated and their family members. Both fiscal and political support could also be bolstered by patient support groups for the diseases and conditions: post-traumatic stress disorder, alcoholism and addiction, depression, neuroses and psychoses, cluster and migraine headaches, obsessive-compulsive disorder, relationship issues, death anxiety, and autism.*

---

*Chapters on all these except autism are in the two-volume set *Psychedelic Medicine* (Winkelman and Roberts 2007). Two autism review articles are Mogar and Aldrich's 1969 "The Use of Psychedelic Agents with Autistic Schizophrenic Children" and Rhead's 1977 "The Use of Psychedelic Drugs in the Treatment of Severely Disturbed Children"). The website "LSD Studies with Autistic Children" (www.neurodiversity.com/lsd.html) contains many of the original, but now dated, articles. But the evidence for treating autism is weaker than for other indications. This is a prime area the proceeds from CPC's IPO could fund. An early research survey on Asperger's syndrome with adults may provide leads.

VC: How long would it take CPC to reach significant milestones?

TR: Actually, in comparison to other start-up pharmaceutical, medical treatment, and biotech companies, several developmental stages have already been completed, and other stages appear just down the road. For example, searching for drug candidates takes years, many false starts, and lots of expensive screening, whereas in relation to this proposal, there are already a dozen or more likely candidates with some history of use and others with pilot studies already completed. These milestones have already been passed even before the company is formed.

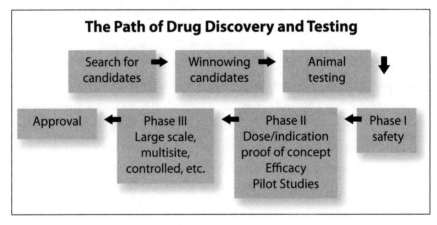

Figure 13.1. The seven stages from drug discovery to final approval

Phase I: Extensive research has already been done on the safety of many of these drug candidates, sometimes under the aegis of research on drugs of abuse and more recently by the movement of psychedelic research into mainstream medical research.

Phase II: Testing of doses for various conditions takes years more, and here too, CPC would be advanced as some of its candidates for investigational new drugs have already been tested for safety, and federal agencies have approved some of them for medical research. For example, work with LSD done in the 1950s, '60s, and '70s has explored and identified various likely uses and treatment protocols. For FDA approval, much of this work would have to be replicated with bigger samples, but again, older preliminary, groundbreaking studies point the way for larger and more carefully controlled clinical studies up to today's standards. Additionally, current clinical research studies provide data about what works and how to increase effectiveness. To investors this is all music to their financial ears: these already completed and in-process tasks reduce CPC's expenses compared with other medical-treatment start-ups and will likely speed bringing CPC to profitability.

Phase III: Much of the money raised by this public offering will be used for Phase III efficacy studies. CPC will use its funds to pay for research at medical research institutes, clinical project sites, and hospitals. The diagram above of the path from drug discovery to approval shows that a huge amount of research has already been accomplished below the radar.

Other markers of progress include governmental approvals for various stages in research, development, production, and treatment, and as noted there is good reason to believe these will be forthcoming because they are consistent with previous decisions. Here again, we are talking about approvals in both the United States and in other countries. Obtaining use patents is another range of systematic advances. To investors, a big advantage of CPC as an investment is that so much has already been achieved.

VC: Wouldn't stockholders support CPC and related drug policies too?

TR: Absolutely. *This should not be underestimated.* It would help a lot to have, say, JPMorganChase Bank, Citicorp, Fidelity, Vanguard, Prudential, Merrill Lynch, and innumerable hedge funds interested in CPC's welfare. These are powerful interests, and they are ones many influential people take seriously. These organizations and substantial individual investors would, in effect, be part of a pro-psychedelics lobby too.

For example, with XYZ National Bank and some of its major stockholders also being stockholders of CPC as well as contributors to political campaign funds, senators and representatives from XYZ's district are going to know where their interests lie. For legislators and regulators, it is one thing to have Dr. X, who has no political clout, apply for permission to do exploratory research on LSD, and it's quite another thing to have a billion-dollar corporation with a network of powerful friends and informed professionals apply. Actually, CPC may very well fund Dr. X's research so that both can benefit.

VC: Why a corporation? There are other ways of using psychedelics and benefiting from them too.

TR: Yes, there are, and they should all be pursued. I am not suggesting that a company like CPC is the only way, but one among others. A whole set of organizations is needed, and the very existence of each will support the others. These would include professional and scholarly organizations, foundations, educational programs, religious groups, and so on.

The history of the development of Fast ForWord illustrates the particular value of forming a corporation, however. When Ed Taub, behavioral neuroscientist on the faculty at the University of Alabama at Birmingham, expressed frustration about how slow the rehabilitation community was to embrace constraint-induced movement therapy for stroke, Michael Merzenich, professor emeritus neuroscientist at the University of California, San Francisco, responded that only the profit motive was strong enough to overcome entrenched professional interests and prejudice. Merzenich told colleagues that forming a business was the only way to get the benefits of neuroplasticity out of the lab and into the hands—or brains, actually—of the people it could help. By October 1996 Merzenich and his partners had secured venture capital funding from E. M. Warberg, and the next month their business, Scientific Learning, conducted its first public demonstration of Fast ForWord at the annual meeting of the American Speech-Language-Hearing Association. "No one would be using Fast ForWord if there were not a commercial force driving it into the world," Merzenich said four years later. "The nonprofit motive is simply too slow" (Jeffrey M. Schwartz and Sharon Begley 2003, 234).

One of the real advantages of a corporation is that it forms a structure for combining the interests and resources of many people into one coordinated crowdfunding effort. There is a lot of good individual work centered around psychedelics, such as books being written and websites produced, and some small-group efforts such as conferences and publications, but a move to an international stage requires the cooperation of thousands of people and coordination among them. Not only does a stock corporation provide a way to collect power and focus energy, but, as a potential profit-making entity, it can recruit people who want to make money, along with their resources and support.

VC: What about all the anti-psychedelic publicity? Wouldn't the word *psychedelic* scare away investors?

TR: I think publicity would come in three phases. First would come the immediate surprised, skeptical, and humorous reactions. Suppose Community Psychedelic Centers International had LSDD as its NASDAQ trading symbol; headline writers would have a field day:

THE SIXTIES REBORN—HEY, MAN, WANT TO BUY SOME LSDD?

or

HEADS UP ON WALL STREET MARKET HIGH ON LSDD HIPPIE INVESTMENT VEHICLE

This is to be expected; it will have the benefit of attracting attention, and it will lead people to examine both the therapeutic research base and CPC's financials and business plan.

A second headline/publicity phase—reflecting interest in and investigation of the claims of CPC's prospectus—would probably tone down the first with views like:

LSD FOR DRUNKS? CPC SAYS IT DRIES THEM OUT

or

INVESTMENT BANKERS TAKING LSD—SERIOUSLY

Perhaps this is more hope than actuality, but I think a third phase is a realistic possibility:

STRONG PREMARKET INDICATIONS CAUSE CPC TO RAISE OFFERING PRICE, NUMBER OF SHARES

or

TODAY'S IPOS—LSDD TAKES INVESTORS HIGHER

The appendix offers a hypothetical "Prospectus" for CPC, which lays out the possibilities in more detail.

14

It Means Something Different to Be Well Educated

When our view of our mind changes, our view of its development changes too. This chapter presents some of the changes that multistate theory offers education. First, we will consider how standard educational topics expand to include our minds' multistate capacities. Then we'll pick up the multistate trail of practices for classrooms and other educational venues. Some speculations on how psychedelics might fit into this picture will follow, and finally, we'll propose a number of innovations in higher education.

HOW DOES EDUCATION CHANGE FROM MINDBODY STATE TO MINDBODY STATE?

The first, broader approach observes that the major topics in education and their foundational questions are usually approached from a single-state perspective, but each psychotechnology and its respective mindbody state recasts those topics and their questions from its perspective. In a second approach, the central multistate research question elaborates the broader topics.

Revisioning the Fields of Educational Studies

In addition to inserting all the questions of education and psychology into the central multistate question, another way to envision educational studies is to ask how each psychotechnology can expand educational topics. For example, what are the effects and implications of, say, various kinds of meditation or biofeedback for what people can learn, for the goals of education, or for how developmental stages interact with psychotechnologies?

Any one of the boxes in this matrix unpacks into an agenda of sub-questions. Addressing each can occupy several professional lifetimes of educational researchers. See the chart on page 209.

Central Multistate Question

This more focused approach recasts fundamental education questions: How do learning, reading, calculating, memory, performances, and so forth vary from state to state? As we move from one mindbody state to another, do we discover not only that these skills become weaker in some states and stronger in others but also that other varieties of them exist? Musicians, actors, dancers, and other performers know what it is like to "be in the zone" for peak performance. During these peaks people typically feel they become one with their performance. They forget time, and the place they are performing often fades away. Changes in identity such as weakened self-identity, timelessness, and focused attention are typical markers of changes in mindbody states. Can we teach people to get "in the zone"? Probably; good actors often learn to slip into a role, and athletic coaches give pep talks before a game or during half-time, which focus their players' attention.

CLASSROOM APPLICATIONS

As the examples in the chapter on enhancing cognition (chapter 9) showed, insights and practical problem solving can take place in other mindbody states. The examples there related to the use of psychedelics. These psychotechnologies clearly are not appropriate for children and

REVISIONING THE MAJOR FIELDS OF EDUCATIONAL STUDIES

Mindbody Psychotechnology	What can be learned/known?	What goals, objectives, and standards?	How do age/stage affect these?	How to assess, evaluate, measure?	What methods teach these?	What place in the curriculum?	How do ethnic/other groups vary?	Implications for gifted/disabled, etc.?
Psychoactive Drugs								
Meditations(s)								
Martial Arts/Yoga								
Hypnosis								
Dreams								
Relaxation/Imagery								
Biofeedback								
Contemplative Prayer								
Sensory Isolation								
Sensory Overload								
Breathing Exercises								

classroom practices, but psychedelics are just one group among many psychotechnologies, many of which can lead to increased learning and problem solving.

Sleeping and dreaming may be the most open avenue to introduce multistate learning. An example of this happened to me when I was a sophomore in high school. Mr. Ebner, my geometry teacher, liked to give us "puzzlers" to work on. One day he gave us this problem: given the three angles of a triangle, but no sides, and the radius of a circle, construct a triangle inscribed in a circle. I thought about it, and thought about it, and thought about it, but could not come up with an answer, so I went to bed with the problem still floating around in the back of my mind. About 2 a.m. I woke up. I had the answer. Although I did not recognize it at the time, this was an early clue to multistate thinking. There is nothing unusual about solving a problem while asleep or while dreaming. "Sleeping on it" is a common multistate psychotechnology.

Can we teach about dreams in schools, not only as something we do but also to provide guidance in using them? Dreaming is an easy first step in developing mindbody skills and a step toward introducing the bigger idea that other mindbody states can be useful.

Do You Have Your Dream for English?

Dreams are also a way to teach students to understand the poetic and symbolic use of words. Early in my career an experienced high school English teacher who was taking my educational psychology class for a master's-level degree wrote a wonderfully titled paper "Do You Have Your Dream for English?" (Hayes 1975). For years she had tried to teach her high school sophomores about the expressive and symbolic uses of language. This did not make much sense to her students, she said, and seemed like a waste of time for her class, but it was part of the syllabus. One day, as a class assignment for me when we were studying the educational uses of humanistic and transpersonal psychologies, she gave her students the assignment of remembering a dream and keeping it in mind for the next day's class. To generate a bit of mystery, she didn't say why. The next day, as she entered her classroom, she heard one student ask another, "Do you have your dream for English?"

She asked them to take out a piece of paper and something to write with, but to temporarily place them toward the corners of their desks. Then she turned out the lights, closed the shades, and told them to put their heads down on their arms for a few minutes. "Now, rerun the dream through your mind and try to re-experience it. Keep re-running it. Remember as many details as you can, and pay attention to how you felt and what you thought."

After several minutes, she said, "Now write your dream on your paper, and be sure to include what happened, what you felt, and what you thought. . . . Write down as much of the dream as you can, and use vivid words and sharp details that express how your dream felt. If you do not know how to spell a word, do the best you can. You won't be graded on this." At the end of the class, she collected the papers saying, "We'll use these tomorrow."

The next day she handed back the papers and instructed them to write poems using the most vivid images, strongest feelings, and expressive vocabulary from the previous day's papers, and "Don't try to make them rhyme. Just make them powerful." This was her introduction to a unit on poetry and became the basis for discussing the symbolic and expressive use of words. Later she wrote:

> The assignment, I felt, was a success for three major reasons: (1) Everyone had something to write about. (2) They were all fascinated by dreams and uninhibited about sharing them. (3) The vivid quality of dreams lends itself to poetic expression.
>
> It was the best first experience in poetry that I have ever tried. (Hayes 1975, 420)

Unintentionally, this was also a beginning lesson in multistate education. It helped the students learn that other mindbody states contain useful ways of thinking, and that people, especially poets and other creative people, use them beneficially to enrich our culture.

THE SAD FATE OF HUMANISTIC EDUCATION

In the 1970s one of multistate education's ancestors tried a wider range of new teaching and learning methods. Some of them are what we would now call mindbody educational methods. Practices and ideas were collected in books such as *The Centering Book* by Gay Hendricks and Russel Wills and *The Second Centering Book* by Gay Hendricks and me. The latter includes a ninety-nine-page topical bibliography of mindbody topics such as dreams, biofeedback, hypnosis, meditation, yoga, and relaxation. The then burgeoning field was attracting innovative educators both in schools and outside them.

At this time, psychology was breaking out of the mold of behaviorism. Cognitive psychologists faulted psychology for omitting higher-level thinking. "How much could we learn about human thinking from studying rats, cats, and guinea pigs?" they asked. "Not much," they answered. This gave birth to cognitive psychology, which now dominates psychology. From a multistate perspective, of course, cognitive psychology also needs to consider cognition in all mindbody states, not just our usual awake state, but most cognitive psychologists are single-state bound.

A second reaction to behavioral psychology raised a parallel criticism. Rather than deriving findings primarily from rat experiments, another group of psychologists, including Abraham Maslow, wanted psychology to pay attention to characteristically human behavior and experience, to become human-based rather than rodent-based, *humanistic* not *rodentistic*. Unfortunately, religious zealots knew only religious meanings for the word *humanistic:* the philosophical stance that there is nothing supernatural, that God does not exist, or, for example, that Jesus was a wise human with wise teaching, but not supernatural in any sense. Humanistic education (not to be confused with the humanities) incensed them. Confusing their meaning of *humanistic* with its meaning in psychology and education, they took off on a crusade against human-based psychology and humanistic education in schools and smothered it. That languages, literature, and philosophy were the humanities and also *humanistic* studies did not deter them from generating a storm cloud of self-righteous anger rooted largely in ignorance about humanistic educational psychology, rather than examining their own mistaken assumptions.

EDUCATION FOR PUBLIC POLICY, WONDER, AND AWE

In *Ayahuasca, Enthogenic Education and Public Policy*, his 2011 dissertation from the University of British Columbia, Kenneth W. Tupper uses a sociohistorical view of the development of cognition in cultures (presumably recapitulated in individuals) as progressing along five stages, each with its respective type of cognition (adapted from Egan 1997).

1. Body-centered and sensory awareness practices
2. Orality and storytelling
3. Literacy, numeracy, and symbolism
4. Logic and rationality
5. Theoretical self-reflexivity

Tupper claims that modern societies and schooling largely neglect the development of the first two stages and their respective somatic and mythic kinds of thinking. This lack reduces our sense of wonder and awe. Tupper contends that entheogens such as ayahuasca are archaic but powerful cognitive tools that can help foster these more primordial forms of cognition and educationally complement the other higher types of cognition. Public policies in both education and drugs need to be reformed from this perspective too, he claims.

According to one of Tupper's earlier articles in the *Journal of Drug Education and Awareness* (2003), traditional indigenous entheogenic practices are a model for the educational deployment of psychoactive substances as cognitive tools. In a more contemporary context, older youth or young adults who are psychologically prepared and screened would be introduced to entheogens through rites of passage and processes of intergenerational education (i.e., elders modeling optimally beneficial use).

A METHOD FOR INVENTING PARADIGMS

In higher education the central multistate question—"How does _____ vary from mindbody state to mindbody state?"—divides into two approaches. The first examines the topics inserted into the question. These are the things we normally explore. For example, "How does memory vary from one state to another?" Using this approach, researchers would look in other states for 1) changes in memory strength and 2) analogs of our default state's memory.

The second approach steps back to get a broader perspective and asks, "How might varying researchers' own mindbody states provide a fresh perspective on a whole field of inquiry and possibly reformulate it?" Psychedelics and other psychotechnologies can be used as conceptual research methods to think outside the box, to reexamine theories, models, paradigms, assumptions, and even our thinking processes. These all become variables.

A personal note: I think our ordinary state and its cognitive processes have evolved for very good reasons. I am quite a fan of our default state. Although ideas in other states may seem insightful and profound at the moment, those inspirational, noetic feelings are not convincing in themselves. William James's "Hogamous Higamous" anecdote is fair warning. Fruitful ideas occur in lots of mindbody states; so do fruitless ones.

Discovering Parameters

To my knowledge, Benny Shanon's 2002 *The Antipodes of the Mind* offers the most fruitful example of this multistate exploration for higher education. His work of combining ayahuasca and cognitive studies shows the richness of stepping back and examining a field of inquiry from a different mindbody perspective. By combining cognitive psychology with mindbody anthropology, he uses ayahuasca experiences to examine cognitive psychology's set of parameters about the human mind. His focus is not on the particular topics of cognitive psychology, but on its unstated assumptions. He asks, in effect, "How does ayahuasca change our perspective on cognitive psychology as a field of study? How do basic assumptions of the field shift?"

In chapter 2 we previewed three of the eleven parameter shifters that Shanon spotted. While each is important, their combined impact is most important. They show how universities, institutes, departments, and programs that promote new visions of disciplines have the potential to 1) identify otherwise unrecognized current assumptions of their fields or 2) reconstruct the foundational assumptions of those disciplines to invent new models of their fields. Following are Shanon's discoveries that expand our current assumptions about how we think about our minds (2002, 198–206).

- Agenthood—experiencing thoughts as not being one's own
- Personal identity—personal identification with whatever one is looking at, a sense of unity with the other
- Unity—being oneself at the same time as being someone or something else
- Boundaries—erasing the boundary between inner and outer reality
- Individuation—self-transcendence but with consciousness still maintained
- Calibration—change in perceptions of one's size, weight, posture, and so on
- Locus of consciousness—consciousness located outside one's physical body
- Time—variations in time, including its speed or even feelings of eternity
- Self-consciousness—a "residue" of the normal self after other facets of consciousness are completely altered

- Intentionality—no object to which thought is being directed and no content entertained by the mind, often leading to a sense of "the Void" or "pure consciousness"
- Connectedness, knowledge, and the conferral of reality—a noetic feeling that one is privy to true knowledge

Inventing Paradigms

Shanon's approach does not just ask questions about established concepts within existing disciplinary models. Most important, his research model offers a systematic method for evolving new paradigms. Anomalies—things that are not supposed to happen according to current theories—are the exceptions that engender new ways of thinking, and other mindbody states often produce anomalies. We no longer have to sit around and wait for enough anomalies to occur to precipitate a crisis within a discipline. In chapter 2, Humanity's Taproot, we saw that mystical experiences are one set of paradigm busters. What other mindbody psychotechnologies and states demand similar reframing?

MULTISTATE PROJECTS FOR HIGHER EDUCATION

Universities or other institutions that take on multistate projects may well build new intellectual endeavors. It would take more than one large university to chase down even the hottest leads, so if multistate models catch on, it is likely that a variety of institutes, centers, and programs will specialize in one or another aspect of multistate research and the new paradigms that unfold. The beginnings are already underway. Some medical schools are investigating meditation, others imagery, and others biofeedback and neurofeedback. Unfortunately, colleges of education and educational foundations shy away from looking at ways to expand educational topics, like those shown in the table Revisioning the Major Fields of Educational Studies on page 209.

Academic disciplines could well organize, for example, a center for mindbody studies in philosophy or an intercultural program for the anthropological study of psychotechnologies. A center of the arts might specialize in how mindbody states can influence the arts, how they already have done so, and how to express and produce mindbody shifts. Almost across the curricula, the sciences, humanities, and the arts can seize wide-open opportunities. Of course, specialized courses in medicine, law, public policy, religious studies, and similar schools are naturals too.

A particularly powerful approach at a university would be to set up an institute with a combination of its own faculty and administration with joint appointments and visiting faculty from existing departments. Alternately, a program in mindbody studies might offer its own courses and include courses from other departments in its curricula.

A historical parallel of this comes from cognitive studies. As the field got off the ground, its early students took courses in contributing disciplines, always asking what that discipline had to say about human thinking. These disciplines often included departments of psychology, philosophy, biology, anthropology, linguistics, and computer technology. Over the years, as graduate students hybridized information from these fields, enriched approaches emerged. Given the interdisciplinary richness of mindbody studies, a similar approach to hybridizing disciplines and methods can produce multistate programs.

Eventually, where are psychedelic and mindbody studies likely to lead higher education? Each year that I offer my class Foundations of Psychedelic Studies I receive inquiries both nationally and internationally from students who want to enroll online. Psychedelic and mindbody topics are perfect candidates for the booming field of massive open online courses. Courses offered online now enroll tens of thousands of students, mostly in technical fields. Major universities are getting into the globalization act, including Stanford, Penn, Michigan, MIT, Princeton, and others. A small beginning would be to offer one psychedelics course per academic department (see figure 1.1 on page 11). Some, such as biology and medicine, have multiple specialties. As this book shows, the humanities such as philosophy and critical studies of films and literature deserve their places too. Politics needs good perinatal analysis as do the other social sciences.

When we expand beyond psychedelic studies to full mindbody studies, the possibilities of a multistate curriculum multiply. It's likely that various types of meditation, biofeedback, martial arts, and other mindbody psychotechnologies will also enrich all the disciplines shown in figure 1.1 on page 11. Will innovative universities seize the lead and stake out a promising psychotechnology by offering, say, a psychedelics studies program? Will another university offer a meditation studies program? The best solution is for a department of mindbody studies or, better yet, given the breadth of opportunities and complexities of the topics, a whole college of mindbody studies. To take advantage of existing specialized knowledge and to promote joint interdepartmental appointments and intramural consulting, a college of mindbody studies would be most efficiently located within a large university.

At first funding seems like an insurmountable problem. Corporate ventures offer one source; given the psychedelic and other mindbody interests of the new technology multimillionaires and billionaires (Markoff 2006), funders may already be primed to fund programs, institutes, and centers at universities (*Sacramento Bee* 2012).

SUMMARY

What are the greatest areas of psychedelics' contributions to human welfare? Psychotherapy and medicine clearly are two. Religion, spirituality, and values are certainly others. The performing arts and visual arts are definitely richer. A dozen or more academic disciplines are beginning to benefit. Behind this growth people are coming to recognize something important about the human mind, the professional tool that every discipline uses. As psychiatrist Lawrence Kubie wrote, "A discipline comes of age and a student of that discipline reaches maturity when it becomes possible to recognize, estimate, and allow for their errors of their tools" (1954, 349). Psychedelics and multistate theory help us recognize limits to our current thinking tool, especially its singlestate limitations. Psychedelics and other psychotechnologies move us beyond that. They provide us with a large mental toolbox, rich with mindbody tools.

15

You Teach *What? Where?*

I teach Foundations of Psychedelic Studies at Northern Illinois University. When I tell people this, their reactions range from thinking that I am joking to disbelief, from smiling enthusiasm to frozen-faced scorn, from curiosity to envy. "You mean they let you get away with that?" is a common question in one form or another. In this chapter I'll answer some questions people have asked and add some informal thoughts and suggestions for prospective teachers and students. If you're a professor, I hope these will help you to offer a similar class. If you're a student, I hope you'll be able to find a professor to oversee an independent study.

I am able to teach Psychedelic Studies at Northern not because the university or its community are unique in any sense. Northern Illinois University is not located in a culture of liberalism or experimentation. NIU is located in DeKalb, Illinois, sixty-five miles west of Chicago in corn and soybean country. The machine-made barbed wire industry started here in 1873 when Joseph Glidden figured out he could adapt his wife's coffee grinder into a machine to make barbed wire. Before that, barbed wire had all been handcrafted and was terribly expensive. DeKalb's nickname is "Barb City." Its high school athletes are the Barbs, and around the frieze adorning the entrance to the old high school are the usual figures to represent industry, agriculture, and learning, all surrounded with a ceramic representation of barbed wire. Thanks to this invention, as the manifest destiny of agriculture moved west, the open ranges of the old West became fenced in, while the barbed wire plant employed much of the city until it shut down.

Wurlitzer organs were a booming business too, and many great church, movie house, and concert hall organs got their starts here, but Wurlitzer shut down too. The first large-scale commercial hybridization of seeds—later animals—began at DeKalb Ag (known by its flying corncob insignia). It was DeKalb's flagship industry until it was bought out, traded, and shut down. Northern Illinois University is the major employer now, and we have not shut down yet.

Northern Illinois University is a state school with about 25,000 students (undergraduate and graduate), mid-size for the Midwest. Our "service area" stretches from the western shore of Lake Michigan to the Mississippi River north of Interstate 80 to the Wisconsin border; it is bigger than Connecticut and includes the glories of Chicago and Cook County, prosperous suburbs, and numerous "Puttyvilles" (the houses in new real estate developments, which are mostly various shades of putty). Geographically our domain is mostly declining factory cities, rural cities, small towns and villages, and square-mile after square-mile of soybeans and corn. NIU is not noted as a hotbed of innovation in higher education, so it seems odd for a course in psychedelics to arise in corn country, but it did.

HINTS TO PROFS

Lesson 1: You Can Do It

When I speak at conferences there is often is someone who hangs around after the usual questions, wistfully saying, "I wish I could teach a course or a unit on psychedelics." My answer is, "You can, especially now. If I can teach a course about psychedelics at Northern Illinois University, you can probably teach one at College X or University Y." Of course, just as psychedelic research has to meet the standards of institutional review boards and the appropriate governmental agencies, a proposal for a new course has to meet the standards of the given college or university.

Compared to 1981, when I started, responsible research is now being recognized. It is hard for a curriculum committee to deny that the topic has been rehabilitated if the proposed bibliography includes the six articles featured in chapter 1, those from the *Lancet, Scientific American,* the *Chronicle of Higher Education,* the *Economist,* the *(APA) Monitor,* and the *New York Times.*

Academicians thrive on good questions, so you may want to approach your curriculum committees by citing these sources, then phrasing a question, "What are the implications of psychedelics for _____? This special topics seminar will examine this question." It's hard to just say "no" to a scholarly or scientific inquiry. Since 1981 the literature on psychedelics has grown in amount and strengthened in quality, as many of the references in this book illustrate.

Lesson 2: Don't Get on Your High Horse

In the early 1980s there was a good balance in the College of Education, where I taught, between the classes that "needed to be covered" and the available professors, and there was a sense of innovation in the air. Professors could offer classes in their specialties if enough students would sign up. This fit my interest in psychedelics, so I proposed a one-off special topics course, Psychedelic Research, and my department head approved it. After all, it was not really adding the course to our curriculum; it was just a one-time offering, or so it seemed at the time. To announce/advertise a course, it was necessary to put up posters around campus, and as I did so, I saw hallways, bulletin boards, and classrooms I never knew existed.

A couple days after I put up the notices, my assistant department chairman asked me to stop by his office. "The assistant provost," he said, "called and wanted to know whether psychedelics were a proper topic for a course." Zoom went my adrenaline. I rushed back to my office and dashed off a letter to the assistant provost saying that I did not think his job description included censoring course content, that university policy and practice was that course content was the prerogative of each department, and that if he disagreed, I offered to discuss the topic at an open meeting of the university council, one of our major governing bodies. By a bit of good luck, the paperback edition of *Psychedelic Drugs Reconsidered* (Grinspoon and Bakalar 1979) had just come out with its splendid forty-page annotated bibliography. I photocopied it and sent it along as evidence of respectable scholarly and scientific work in psychedelics. Two days later my assistant department chair let me know that the assistant provost had called again to say that he had inquired "because someone had asked."

Since then I have mellowed about criticism, real or imagined. At least I like to think I have; there has not been any explicit criticism that I know of. Now I try to recognize that people who question or criticize the course do so from a responsible perspective of caring for student welfare and for keeping them away from "drugs that rot people's minds." These challenges, if they arise, are teachable moments. They present a chance to inform well-meaning, honestly concerned people about both psychedelics' realistic dangers and their evidence-based benefits.

If you run into a similar situation, I recommend acknowledging the other person's real concerns (at least to yourself) and taking him or her one step toward a balanced view of psychedelics. When approaching someone who is not up to date on the new research on psychedelics, it works best to give or send them only one brief item such as the article in the *Lancet* or the one in *Scientific American;* people are more likely to read one brief item but lay aside a thick batch of readings. Do not overwhelm them; teach them.

Many of us do not change our minds quickly. It may take two or three exposures to new information before it starts to look credible. The exposure you provide may be number one, so do not push things. You do not want to force your "student" to resist your efforts and then reject exposures two and three. By exposure three, he or she may begin to think, "This feels familiar" and suspect, "Maybe there is something to this after all."

Lesson 3: You May Have Hidden Allies
The few people I know who have started to teach about psychedelics either as a full course or as a unit within another course ran into

surprisingly little opposition and—even more surprising to them—apparent support from higher ups where they had not anticipated it. Instead of running into supposed obstacles, my "psychedelic colleagues" report comments like "I was a student during the '60s" and "It is time we reopened research about this topic" or "I remember reading some promising research about this when I was a student." These statements seemed to indicate more than academic open-mindedness, more like veiled enthusiasm.

Considering that official government statistics estimate that more than 23 million people in the United States have dropped acid, it is not surprising that some of them are now colleagues or in administrative and other leadership positions in higher education. Maybe that guy sitting in the dean's chair is a former acidhead with fond memories and unanswered questions.

CLASS NOTES

Rather than describe my syllabus, which progresses from year to year, I have placed it online: niu.academia.edu/ThomasRoberts. Following are a few additional classroom hints.

Discussions

My class is a seminar of fifteen honors students who are juniors or seniors, so there is time for class discussions. After announcements and similar introductory material, I like to begin each session by asking the students what questions and comments they have on that day's readings. For many of them it is the smallest class they have had, and they are shy about talking in class. They are afraid somebody "will jump down my throat," that is, strongly, even rudely, disagree with them. To set the tone and expectation for daily discussions, in the first class I pair them up and, after a few minutes of chatting with their partners, have them introduce their partners to the class, including an accomplishment their partner is proud of. By the end of the first class everyone has spoken and probably made a new acquaintance. This usually breaks the ice.

Internet Field Trips

The "Internet Field Trips" for the class come in two types. One is weekly assigned visits with the question "What did you find of interest at the site?" The chosen sites are the best psychedelic reference resources. While calling them "field trips" is only a cognitive reframing, it works better than calling them "assignments." The other type is that of taking recommended, recreational field trips for the fun of it, and to answer the question "Can you find something of value for our class?" Thanks to the Internet age, there are thousands of websites, and the student age cohort likes surfing around from site to site. Often students find YouTube and other sites that are worth telling the class about and which are shared in the syllabus for future classes.

Self-selected Books

One of the enjoyable things about the class is that the students come from all majors across the university, and by the time they are juniors and seniors they are able to bring some of the ideas from their home disciplines to class. Sometimes this will show up in the choice of a self-selected book. They may want to read, say, about sociology or biochemicals and psychedelics. I like them to be able to link academic topics, and with the permission of another professor they may write a combined paper for my psychedelics course and for another course. In "Multidisciplinary Approaches to Psychedelic Scholarship," I've given some ideas of how undergraduates can work psychedelics into their classes and programs. Sometimes this alerts the professors in other courses about some psychedelic aspects of their disciplines. Other students use their self-selected book to explore an area new to them. I pass around books from my own collection to give them other ideas.

Typically, of fifteen students two may have had some experience with psychedelics, so first-person accounts such as Charles Hayes' *Tripping* appeal for that reason. If a book is especially weighty, such as Shanon's *Antipodes of the Mind,* two students may do a joint report.

Why Not to Put LSD in Your Friend's Coffee

If I read my students correctly, the few who come to the class as enthusiastic evangelists for psychedelics for everyone become much more circumspect as the class progresses. The case studies in Stan Grof's *LSD: Doorway to the Numinous* (2009) help them become aware of psychological difficulties that lie hidden in everyone's mind, their own as well as their friends'. The "coffee lecture" is one of my first lectures. The gist of it is in the box below. Afterward I expect my students to be able to list "the reasons not to" and summarize them for a quiz. When we discuss current research such as the Johns Hopkins studies, I remind them that the results came from volunteers who were carefully selected, thoroughly prepared, accompanied during sessions, and helped to integrate their experiences afterward. This is the way research, treatment, and experiences should be conducted.

Why You Shouldn't Put LSD in Your Friend's Coffee

- The drug you buy from a dealer may not actually be the drug you want; some dealers will sell you anything and tell you it's what you want. Also, the dose will be unknown, and it may be contaminated with other drugs or who-knows-what. Unfortunately, this danger is largely a result of our current drug policies.

- Psychedelics can activate parts of the unconscious mind that cause great anxiety and should be faced only in the company of a qualified therapist. These might include traumatic experiences, for example, or childhood fears. Stan Grof's work gives examples of this; fortunately, his patients were undergoing psychedelic psychotherapy, not taking the drug on their own. For someone who is prepsychotic, a psychedelic could cause a bad trip or even tip the balance into psychosis. In normal people also, a psychedelic can bring up irrational fears and thoughts that can continue to interfere with their lives after the drug is gone.

- People have idiosyncratic reactions to drugs. Some people are allergic to aspirin, others to antibiotics. Genetic differences probably play a role too. For example, Ecstasy (MDMA) works by flooding the space between cells (the synapse) with serotonin. Serotonin is then carried back to the cells by "transporter proteins" to be reused. Some Ecstasy users are prone to depression because they have a short version of the gene that produces a less efficient transporter. People with two short genes are even more susceptible to depression after MDMA. As the field of pharmacogenomics—the study of the interactions between genes and drugs—grows, it's likely that other gene-based drug effects will be discovered. You don't know about your friend's possible reactions to an unknown drug, and your friend probably doesn't know either.

- If your friend is pregnant, psychedelics can instigate a miscarriage by causing uterine contractions. According to Grof's work, if a woman re-experiences her own birth during the perinatal stage, this sometimes includes uterine contractions.

- Grof makes a sensitive psychiatric point: although the myth of psychedelics causing birth defects is fading away, a certain number of babies are born with defects even to mothers who have had excellent prenatal care. If this happens to a mother who did psychedelics when she was pregnant—even though she knows the birth defect rumor is a myth—she may think every day for the rest of her life, "What if I hadn't?"

- Should you slip a dose into your friend's coffee? If you believe, as I do, that each person has the right to determine what goes on in his or her own mind, then putting a drug in your friend's coffee destroys this freedom. You are infringing this right to mental self-control.

Source: From the syllabus for the course Foundations of Psychedelic Studies at Northern Illinois University.

Guest Speakers

Maybe I have just been lucky, but most semesters we have enjoyed speakers two or more times. For example, Dr. Nicholas Cozzi, whose course at University of Wisconsin School of Medicine and Health is mentioned below, covers the rudiments of chemical structure, neurotransmitters, and receptors. Two Native Americans have presented aspects of peyote medicine. Bruce Sewick, who teaches Psychedelic Mindview at the nearby College of DuPage, connects drug policy and mental health policies. Most recently Stephan Beyer, author of *Singing to the Plants* (2010), introduced students to the current hot topic of ayahuasca. Each speaker brings his own scholarly flavor to psychedelic scholarship, enriching it beyond my perspective.

Don't Ask, Don't Tell

In the syllabus there is a boxed paragraph, "Psychedelic Warning Label." At the first class meeting I point this out and tell the students that although I will talk about my psychedelic experiences, I am not modeling behavior that I expect them to follow. Communication in our class is not privileged as it would be with a doctor, clergy member, or lawyer, so they may want to shade their own experiences with "someone I know," "I heard that," "one of my friends says," and so forth. Sometimes smirks speak louder than words.

HIGHER HIGHER EDUCATION

One reason I started my course was my hope that if I could teach it at Northern Illinois University, it would be an ice-breaker for professors elsewhere. Until the past three or four years, I was disappointed, but now that a more rational, evidence-based approach to psychedelics is spreading in both science and society, hope blooms again. At College of DuPage, a community college in suburban Chicago, Psychedelic Mindview is geared toward people in the human services field like mental health professionals and addiction counselors. Psychedelics: Theory, Research, and Clinical Applications at Sofia University in Palo Alto, California, is primarily for graduate students who plan to become mental health professionals.

Bellevue Hospital–NYU Medical School is the world leader in psychedelic medical education. There, doctors Stephen Ross and Jeffrey Guss teach Psychedelics in Psychiatry. In case there is any doubt about the range of professionals who are interested in psychedelics, Dr. Guss describes their students this way:

> The class was open to a broad variety of individuals. We invited the Fellows in Addiction Psychiatry in the NYU Department of Psychiatry, and there was one senior resident (PGY-IV) who was doing a selective in PRG (the research program that is doing the psilocybin/cancer anxiety research, Psychedelic Research Group). In addition we invited people from a diverse group of professional categories who had expressed an interest in our research. There were doctoral students in psychology from the New School, as well as NYU, doctoral students in Cognitive Neuroscience, research associates from Ken Alper's ibogaine program, nursing students, social workers involved with addiction treatment and addiction program development, as well as numerous non-clinical individuals (meditation enthusiasts with degrees in consciousness studies), researchers from the Manhattan Veterans Administration, and so forth. (2011, personal communication)

In addition to providing psychotherapy for their patients and testing their hypotheses, the NYU–Bellevue course enriches the general discourse. As a center for bringing together knowledge from the participants' own academic areas and alternative medicine, the course helps students and instructors meet with other like-minded medical and academic professionals to share ideas; ideas about meditation, Buddhism, drumming, and similar mindbody topics cross-fertilize discussions. From an institutional perspective, in addition to familiarizing the participants with the specific treatment protocols and staff, the course is a forum for graduate students at NYU to discuss their personal ideas for research in a supportive environment.

The Midwest is moving forward too. In addition to my course and Bruce Sewick's at the College of DuPage, at the University of Wisconsin School of Medicine and Health, Professor Nicholas Cozzi includes a one-hour lecture on psychedelics in his Integrated Neurosciences course primarily for second-year medical students (2011 personal communication). At the University of Minnesota's Center for Spirituality and Healing, one of Dennis McKenna's courses includes components on psychedelics—People, Plants and Drugs: An Introduction to Ethnopharmacology.

PSYCHEDELIC COURSE DEVELOPMENT PRIZE AWARDS

A high-benefit funding opportunity exists for foundations and wealthy individuals. Colleges and universities take an academic field seriously if grants are available in that field. While funders have been generous in their donations to support research, funding new psychedelics courses would be relatively cheap and long lasting. Once a course is established it can go on for decades. More than that, it lends legitimacy to its topic. Of course this might be done various ways, but I propose that the way to have the biggest impact would be a three-round contest.

ROUND 1: an announcement in *The Chronicle of Higher Education* and elsewhere alerts professors to Psychedelic Course Design Awards. Professors submit letters of intent with brief descriptions of their qualifications and their institution's willingness to support it.

ROUND 2: selected winners of the first round receive $2,000 design grants to write a full course proposal. They design their courses and submit detailed syllabi accompanied by a letter from their department chairs or other administration confirming that, if funded, the course would be offered and otherwise supported. Consistent with institutional policies, courses may be in-classroom, online, or both.

ROUND 3: winning proposals are selected. The writers and their departments are awarded with, say, $20,000 each. The professor's award is a Psychedelic Course Design Prize. The department's award is to help pay for the professor's salary while teaching the course and for overhead expenses.

To increase the impact, stage-three awards might be extended for two or three years, or longer. Besides colleges and universities, specialized institutions of higher education such as medical schools, seminaries, and theological schools, law schools, and similar organizations could be eligible to apply for psychedelic course development prize awards too.

For a professor, winning a prize award looks good on a yearly report of professional activities and on a curriculum vita when applying for a new job. For a department and university, winning a prize award is a "boastable" achievement worthy of a public relations announcement.

SUMMARY

Psychedelic courses are fun to teach. The topic itself weaves together strands from diverse disciplines. Nothing helps a class more than student interest, and many of the students who sign up are curious about the topic. It is one of the hot topics in science and society. New research, books, and websites come along in a steady stream. DVDs, videos, and webcasts proliferate.

Are you thinking of proposing a one-time psychedelics special topics seminar, proposing a cataloged course, or including a psychedelic unit in an existing course? Do it.

Hopes

Authors hope their readers will adopt various ideas, insights, and attitudes from their writing. Here are my hopes for *The Psychedelic Future of the Mind*.

In addition to their uses in psychotherapy I hope you will see the importance of psychedelics for religion, for simplifying and enriching daily life, and for increasing our understanding of the human mind— both our own and others'.

I hope you will savor the rich diet of ideas that produce new flavors of history, philosophy, art and film criticism, all the humanities and arts, and most of the sciences.

If you are an ordinary citizen whose previous perspective on psychedelics was one of fear and loathing, I hope you are more informed and friendly now.

If you are someone who previously thought everyone should do psychedelics and that there is little to worry about in taking them yourself and encouraging others to do so, I hope you have tempered your enthusiasm by realizing that the best current practice is for people to be screened, prepared, accompanied by skilled guides, and debriefed afterward in order to integrate their experiences into insightful ways of feeling, thinking, and living.

If you were unaware of current research, I hope this book has informed you. High-quality new studies appear from time to time, and I hope you will keep informed of them and, better yet, support the research institutions that are doing this research and the public associations that help sponsor it.

If you are a member of a foundation, I hope you will discover how funding psychedelic research can forward your group's goals.

If you are a member of the news media, I hope you will refrain from razzmatazzing your stories. And I hope you will report forthcoming research accurately.

If you are a politician, I hope you will refrain from fear mongering and at the same time recognize both the real dangers and real benefits from psychedelics by writing laws that take both into account.

If you are interested in religion and spiritual development, I hope you will become informed about the mystical traditions of your religion, and, if your mind is willing, of other religions too. I hope you recognize that psychological exploration carried far enough becomes spiritual exploration.

If you are a college professor, I hope you will design and offer a course about the psychedelic possibilities in your discipline or include a psychedelic unit in your courses. I hope you will present psychedelic papers at conferences, influence professional organizations, and join others.

If you are intrigued with the idea of knowing yourself better by exploring your own mind, I hope you will find a way to do so in a safe and legal setting.

If you are a financier or other kind of businessperson, I hope you will help found a company whose service will include all the necessary steps to provide safe psychedelic journeys.

I hope you are less addicted to fame, power, and money and more motivated by knowledge, beauty, humane service, and enlightenment.

I hope you will follow up with the authors and groups that you ran across in this book. They lead the way to future human improvement, both individually and collectively.

I hope you will see psychedelics as part of a richer view of what it means to be a person. They are just one family of psychotechnologies for developing our full human potential. Our default mindbody state is a good one, but we should not remain stuck there.

I hope you will wear your selfness more comfortably and at the same time realize it is not all you are.

I hope each chapter will jostle your mind into sprouting new ideas.

APPENDIX

Community Psychedelic
Centers International, Inc.

NOTES FOR A PROSPECTUS

PRELIMINARY PROSPECTUS

Community Psychedelic Centers International, Inc.
Incorporated in the State of Delaware

An offering of 50,000,000 shares of common stock at $20 each

SUMMARY Community Psychedelic Centers International, Inc. ("CPC" or "the company") anticipates offering 50,000,000 shares of common stock on or about (date forthcoming). This will be the initial public offering for the company and may represent special risks. The company expects to provide two types of services: (1) psychedelic-assisted psychotherapy and (2) and psychedelic-assisted professional development. With the proceeds of this offering, the company expects to establish therapeutic centers and professional development centers. The therapeutic centers will consist of (1) free-standing, self-contained centers for referral patients and (2) on-grounds, in-house centers located at existing major mental health hospitals and centers. The professional development centers will provide service for clients who wish to enhance religious experience, creativity, personal growth, academic and scholarly research, and similar non-therapeutic purposes.

The company believes it has already identified several potential drug candidates as investigational drugs, and furthermore, that while additional studies may be required to firmly establish their safety and efficacy, preliminary studies support both.

Underwritten by

HOFMANN & NIEWKRANIUM, INC.
Member of the Zurich, New York, and Amsterdam Stock Exchanges

HANDPIK & QUEST, INC.
Member of the Sausalito, La Honda, and Montauk Stock Exchanges

THE SECURITIES

This offering consists of 50,000,000 shares of common stock in Community Psychedelic Centers International, Inc., (CPC) at an anticipated price of $20 per share.

The securities offered herein represent equal shares of ownership in CPC and currently are not publicly traded, and there can be no assurance that a public market will develop, or if developed, there can be no assurance of market liquidity.

Trading Symbol

Community Psychedelic Centers International has applied to the National Association of Securities Dealers Automated Quotation system (NASDAQ) to trade CPC stock under the symbol LSDD.

Possible Unusual Demand

In addition to the usual financial interest in initial public offerings in the health care industry, CPC believes that indications of interest in CPC stock at its initial public offering may be unusually strong because:

- Some potential investors have experienced psychedelic drugs themselves and believe they have benefited from doing so.
- Some potential investors know people who have experienced psychedelic drugs and believe they have benefited from doing so.
- Some potential investors are familiar with the findings of pilot and preliminary studies (See "The Candidate Drugs" below).
- Some potential investors assume that the processes of drug discovery and preliminary safety and efficacy testing are largely accomplished and will speed the development of CPC.
- During the process of due diligence, individual and institutional investors will examine the evidence for psychedelics' safety and efficacy and will judge them both safe and efficacious when used as the company proposes.

Additionally, CPC recognizes that this offering may attract an unusual amount of media publicity on the Internet, broadcast, and print media, thereby possibly increasing demand for its stock. Accordingly, and depending on demand for the stock, market conditions, and other factors, the price per share, number of shares, or both may be adjusted either up or down. There is no guarantee that any or all of these expectations will be met.

Charitable Allotment

An unusual feature of this offering is the "charitable allotment." Purchasers of these shares at the underwriting are required to donate half their purchases to a charity recognized as such by the United States Internal Revenue Service or by appropriate state, local, or national laws in the jurisdictions where purchasers reside. When considering this requirement, purchasers of shares at the initial public offering may be referred to as "investor-donors." If an investor-donor buys 200 shares, he or she must donate 100 shares to a recognized charity. These shares are fully registered and identical to all other shares. CPC's tax consultants believe that such gifts may qualify as a charitable donation for federal income tax purposes, but the Internal Revenue Service has not made a determination on this issue. Investor-donors should note this additional risk. Investor-donors may select any charity or charities of their choice, such as a church, university, museum, community organization, or other legally recognized eleemosynary institution.

Future Financing

Due to the unpredictable nature of the company's business, additional funding may be necessary in the future. This may be equity, loan, or both. Typically for companies such as CPC, other financings are undertaken as milestones in the companies' plans are reached. There is no assurance that CPC will reach these milestones or that financing will be forthcoming in the future.

THE COMPANY

History

In [month] of [year], CPC Partnership was formed with 20 partners. This partnership organized Community Psychedelic Centers International, Inc. (CPC) and incorporated it in the state of Delaware. CPC has applied to the Food and Drug Administration to commence clinical trials of several drugs which CPC believes offer advantages as adjuncts to psychotherapy. CPC also believes these drugs as used within the confines of the proposed sessions are effective methods of increasing professional development including, but not limited to, creativity and problem solving, providing insights of value to academic and scientific researchers, enhancing primary religious experience, stimulating artistic works, and ways of exploring and developing the human mind. No assurance can be given that the candidate drugs will prove effective, and if they are, no assurance can be given that the FDA will approve their uses as anticipated by CPC.

Unlike pharmaceutical companies, whose business is the manufacture and sale of pharmaceuticals, CPC's primary business will not consist of drug sales, but will consist of the service of providing professionally guided psychedelic sessions. CPC may derive some income from the manufacture and sale of its drugs, but this is expected to be incidental to the company's main business, and CPC expects to derive little, if any, profit from the manufacture and sale of drugs. The company's primary service will include screening and preparation for the sessions, the sessions themselves, and follow-up procedures. These sessions may be for either therapeutic or professional development purposes.

Corporate Structure

The company's structure consists of two divisions, the therapy division and the professional development division. The company calls prospective purchasers of the services of the therapy division "patients," and calls prospective purchasers of the services of the professional development division "clients." Depending on regulatory and other matters, the two divisions and their centers may be located in the same state or in different states and in the same nation or in different nations. (See "Location" below.) They may also be housed together or separately.

CPC CORPORATE DIVISIONS

Therapy Centers

alcoholism
Drug addiction
Post-traumatic stress disorder
Depression
Memory recovery
Boosting immune system
Neuroses and psychoses
Hospice care
Training mental health professionals
Sexual dysfunction
Obsessive-compulsive disorder
Migraine and cluster headaches
Positive psychological health

Professional Development Centers

Spiritual development and religious studies
Creativity and problem solving
Self-development and self-knowledge
Research and education

       Scholarly and academic
       Mental health
       Scientific
       War/peace studies
       Aesthetic

Mapping human mind
Inventing new mindbody states
Constructing new cognitive processes

Therapy Division

The therapy centers will provide services only to clients who are referred by mental health professionals who are certified or licensed in the jurisdictions where the centers are located. In the United States, these will vary from state to state. Internationally, these will vary from country to country. Officially recognized competent authorities are likely to include psychiatrists, clinical psychologists, and others similarly licensed or certified.

At the present, CPC believes its proposed therapeutic services have been shown by preliminary studies to be safe and efficacious for the following indications: alcoholism, drug addiction, post-traumatic stress disorder, lost memory recovery, depression, autism, death anxiety, and selected neurotic and psychotic diagnoses recognized in the *Diagnostic and Statistical Manual*. Regulatory approval will require additional studies to establish these claims.

As experience with these drugs increases and CPC's method of running sessions becomes established, CPC believes that other indications will emerge. Among these is the possibility that intense, overwhelming self-transcendent experiences may boost the immune system. CPC believes that existing studies suggest this may be the case, but that such evidence is not strong, and that additional studies may or may not confirm these leads.

Current plans for the therapy centers call for some of its centers to be located in-house or on the grounds of existing mental health facilities such as state mental hospitals, private residential treatment centers, and similar locations. Other centers will be located as free-standing centers. CPC envisions free-standing centers located to serve the needs of several mental health facilities and professionals in an area.

CPC believes that psychedelic sessions also have value in the training of mental health professionals and will provide both pre-service and in-service education for these groups. CPC plans to apply to appropriate governmental agencies or educational accrediting agencies for permission to offer Continuing Education Units, "CEU's," for this training. In some cases these CEU's may be offered in conjunction with educational institutions such as medical schools, nursing schools, institutions of higher education, professional societies, and others. Here again, standards for national and local jurisdictions will need to be met.

While CPC believes enough referrals will occur to make the therapy centers profitable, no assurance can be given that this will be the case.

Professional Development Division

Professional development centers will provide services for professional and vocational development in business, religion, education, scholarship, science, law, mental health, the arts, and related fields. Instead of being undertaken for the purpose of curing an existing mental health condition, sessions of the professional development centers will be undertaken to work in the fields listed above. CPC believes the proposed services have been shown to be safe and efficacious, but CPC makes no assurance that regulatory agencies will interpret the existing studies this way. A major barrier to regulatory approval is the assumption that psychoactive substances have appropriate use only in medicine and psychotherapy. CPC may have to undertake, or cause to be undertaken, additional studies to provide evidence of the usefulness of psychedelic sessions for non-medical purposes.

Because the proposed activities of the professional development centers are not medical or psychotherapeutic, it is not clear what governmental agencies, if any, have jurisdiction over these issues. This unresolved regulatory issue is especially acute for the religious, artistic, and educational uses because these areas have traditionally been outside U. S. government control. Pending the resolution of this issue, CPC believes that the first professional development centers may be established outside the United States.

Clients of the professional development division must be certified as at low risk of aversive consequences from their sessions, and, like the patients of the therapy centers, they will undergo screening, preparation, the session itself, and post-session follow-up.

Some professional development centers may be associated within one specific institution such as a major university, research facility, church, or monastery; others may serve consortia of institutions; and others may be associated with, or sponsored by, professional organizations. Professional development centers may be owned and operated by CPC or autonomous individuals under license and supervision from CPC.

SESSIONS

Both therapeutic services and professional development services will consist of four phases: (1) screening, (2) preparation, (3) monitoring the session, (4) post-session follow-up. Because these differ according to the nature of the patients and clients and the nature of the desired outcomes, the details of the procedures are only summarized here and are more fully described in *Manual of Procedures for Psychedelic Sessions*, which is incorporated herein by reference.

Screening consists of physical and psychological examinations to determine whether the applicant clients and patients are physically hardy enough to withstand possible emotional and psychosomatic stress. *Preparation* consists of determining the client's/patient's personal preferences of setting and explaining to the client/patient the kinds of experiences he or she is likely to experience during the session, the activities which may occur (such as listening to music), and so forth. It will include establishing rapport with the guide or guides who will attend the patient/client during the session day.

In order to *monitor* a session, which will typically take a full day after a drug has been administered, the client/patient will be accompanied throughout by at least one professional. After a session, which may last twelve hours or more, clients and patients may stay overnight at the center or may be accompanied to their homes. In the case of patients in the therapy centers who are residents at mental health treatment facilities, they will be returned to the custody of their institutions either the same day, or they may stay overnight and return the next day.

During *follow up,* the session and its effects will be evaluated. In the case of patients, this activity will include the patient's doctor or therapist or both. In the case of clients of the professional development centers, the client, as well as the session guide, will typically evaluate the outcome. Due to the nature of psychedelic sessions, the follow-up evaluations may include unanticipated results as well as the intended ones.

REGULATORY MATTERS

Candidate Drugs

The drugs CPC plans to test and develop are psychoactive drugs commonly known as "psychedelic" or "hallucinogenic" drugs. These include, but are not limited to: LSD, DPT, DMT, MDA, MDMA, psilocybin, ayahuasca, ibogaine, and mescaline. Other compounds may be added from time to time. Currently these drugs are Schedule I drugs, meaning they are classified as having strong potential for abuse and no accepted medical value. CPC believes that this scheduling is in error and that these compounds should be listed as Schedule II drugs, meaning they have both recognized medical uses and recognized risks. CPC believes clinical trials have shown these drugs have therapeutic value and can be used safely. CPC will have to expand these trials, including adding more controls. There can be no assurance that CPC will successfully show safety and efficacy, and if successful, there can be no assurance the United States Food and Drug Administration will reclassify them.

CPC believes that these drugs should not be prescribed to patients in such a way that the patients can buy them and self-administer them, but that their proper use requires the presence of fully trained professionals, similar in this respect to the way anesthetics are currently administered. CPC's business will be to provide screening and preparation for the pre-sessions, administration and guidance during the sessions, and follow-up after the sessions.

Drug Discovery

While most pharmaceutical companies and drug discovery companies spend much of their effort identifying new drug candidates, CPC believes it has already identified potentially successful investigational drug candidates, including those listed above. In CPC's view, this may eliminate or reduce both the expense of identifying potential drug candidates and the time needed to identify them.

CPC believes that search, winnowing, animal studies, and Phase I studies are completed or nearly completed for many of its candidate treatment drugs, and Phase II as shown in chapter 13 has been completed for some others.

Drug Testing and Approval

CPC also believes that Phase I safety and Phase II/III efficacy trials can be completed more quickly than is the case with most new investigational drugs because preliminary studies already indicate these drugs can be safely used in an investigational capacity. Because appropriate federal agencies in the United States and in selected foreign countries have already granted some of these drugs the status of investigational drugs, CPC believes its applications for the same status will be approved expeditiously. Building on these pilot and preliminary studies, CPC plans to commence combined Phase I safety trials and Phase II trials to identify possible indications for psychedelic psychotherapy. Here too, CPC believes, preliminary investigations have already identified indications for psychedelics as psychotherapeutic adjuncts. Although CPC believes preliminary identification of investigational new drug candidates has already been achieved, that safety has already been demonstrated, and that pilot studies already indicate likely uses in psychotherapy, there can be no assurance that these goals have been met, and there can be no assurance that United States federal regulatory agencies will share CPC's opinions.

LOCATION

Long-term plans call for CPC to offer its services internationally. While CPC plans to establish therapy centers and professional development centers first within the United States, then internationally, should the regulatory climate prove difficult in the US and more favorable in other nations, this order may be reversed. CPC may even offer its services only in countries other than the United States. CPC will apply for approval by other governments to establish centers in their respective jurisdictions. This possibility includes, but is not limited to, countries in the European Common Market. Because of their histories of successful psychedelic psychotherapy and research, CPC believes that countries with more favorable regulatory climate include Switzerland, the Netherlands, Spain, Germany, Scandinavian countries, and the Czech Republic. Other countries may also be included, and CPC recognizes that Eastern European countries with a need for hard currencies may be especially willing to have CPC develop centers within their borders. These would be available for both nationals of the host countries and for nationals of other countries; the latter, especially if from hard currency countries, would contribute to the economic development of the host countries.

OTHER MATTERS

Insurance and medical coverage: at this time these services are not covered by insurance payments or group health care plans. CPC hopes that as the safety and efficacy of CPC's services become established, insurance plans and national health plans will add psychedelic sessions to their eligible treatments. There can be no assurance they will do so, or if they do so, there can be no assurance that the entire cost of treatment will be covered.

References

"Acid Tests. Research into Hallucinogenic Drugs Begins to Shake Off Decades of Taboo." 2011. The Economist. www.economist.com/node/18864332. Accessed June 23, 2011.

Alfandre, David. 2011. "Physicians Recommend Different Treatment for Patients Than They Would Choose for Themselves." *Archives of Internal Medicine* 171, no. 18: 1,685.

"Anthropologists Find American Heads Are Getting Larger." 2012. Science-Daily. www.sciencedaily.com/releases/2012/05/120530115828.htm. Accessed October 17, 2012.

Armstrong, Karen. 2009. *The Case for God*. New York: Alfred A. Knopf.

Badiner, Allan H. 2002. *Zig Zag Zen: Buddhism and Psychedelics*. San Francisco: Chronicle Books.

Beckley Foundation. www.BeckleyFoundation.org.

Berg, Daniel, Matthew Kirkham, Heng Wang, et al. 2011. "Dopamine Controls Neurogenesis in the Adult Salamander Midbrain in Homeostasis and during Regeneration of Dopamine Neurons." *Cell Stem Cell* 8, no. 4: 426–33.

Beyer, Stephan. 2010. *Singing to the Plants: A Guide to Mestizo Shamanism in the Upper Amazon*. Albuquerque: University of New Mexico Press.

Bourguignon, Erica, ed. 1973. *Religion, Altered States of Consciousness, and Social Change*. Columbus: Ohio State University.

Breitbart, W., C. Gibson, S. R. Poppito, et al. 2004. "Psychotherapeutic Interventions at the End of Life: A Focus on Meaning and Spirituality." *Canadian Journal of Psychiatry* 49: 366–72.

Bromell, Nick. 2000. *Tomorrow Never Knows: Rock and Psychedelics in the 1960s*. New York: Seven Stories Press.

Bronowski, Jacob. 1976. *The Ascent of Man*. Boston: Little Brown & Co. www .brainyquote.com/quotes/quotes/j/jacobbrono149490.html. Accessed May 12, 2012.

Brown, Susan. 2006. "Researchers Explore New Visions for Hallucinogens." The Chronicle of Higher Education, Dec. 8. http://chronicle.com/weekly/v53/ i16/16a01201.htm. Accessed October 16, 2012.

"Buddhism & Psychedelics." 1996. *Tricycle: The Buddhist Review* 6, no. 1: 1–109.

Burnham, Sophy. 1997. *The Ecstatic Journey; The Transforming Power of Mystical Experience*. New York: Ballentine Books.

Campbell, Joseph. 1968. *The Hero with a Thousand Faces*. Princeton: Princeton University Press.

———. 1982. "Envoy: No More Horizons." Chapter 12 in *Myths to Live By*. New York: Bantam.

Caporael, Linnda R. 1976. "Ergotism: The Satan Loosed in Salem?" *Science* 192: 21–26.

Cardena, Etzel, Steven J. Lynn, and Stanley C. Krippner, eds. 2004. *Varieties of Anomalous Experience: Examining the Scientific Evidence*. Washington, D.C.: American Psychological Association.

Cardena, Etzel, and Michael Winkelman, eds. 2011. *Altering Consciousness: Multidisciplinary Perspectives*. 2 vols. Santa Barbara, Calif.: Praeger.

Carman, Aaron, Jeffrey H. Mills, Antje Krenz, et al. 2011. "Adenosine Receptor Signaling Modulates Permeability of the Blood–Brain Barrier." *The Journal of Neuroscience* 31, no. 37: 13272–80.

Cassel, E. J. 1982. "The Nature of Suffering and the Goals of Medicine." *New England Journal of Medicine* 306: 639–45.

Choi, James J., Kirsten Selert, Fotios Vlachos, et al. 2011. "Noninvasive and Localized Neuronal Delivery Using Short Ultrasonic Pulses and Microbubbles." *Proceedings of the National Academy of Sciences, PNAS Early Edition*. www.pnas.org/cgi/doi/10.1073/. Accessed Sept. 20, 2011.

Cohen, S. 1965. "LSD and the Anguish of Dying." *Harper's* September: 69–78.

Committee on Military and Intelligence Methodology for Emergent Neurophysiological and Cognitive/Neural Science Research in the Next Two

Decades. National Research Council of the National Academies. 2008. *Emerging Cognitive Neuroscience and Related Technologies.* Washington, D.C.: The National Academies Press.

Compton, William C., and Edward Hoffman. 2012. *Positive Psychology: The Science of Happiness and Flourishing.* Belmont, Calif.: Wadsworth/Cengage.

"Cool Uses: Alba." GFP: Green Fluorescent Protein. www.conncoll.edu/ccacad/ zimmer/GFP-ww/cooluses8.html. Accessed October 16, 2012.

Corbyn, Zoë. 2011. "How the Penis Lost Its Spikes. Humans Ditched DNA to Evolve Smooth Penises and Bigger Brains." Nature.com. www.nature.com/ news/2011/110309/full/news.2011.148.html. Accessed Mar. 9, 2011.

Cotton, Ian. 1996. "Visions of Heaven and Hell." Chapter 8 in *The Hallelujah Revolution: The Rise of the New Christians.* Amherst, N.Y.: Prometheus Books.

Council on Spiritual Practices. 2011. Johns Hopkins psilocybin studies archive. http://csp.org/psilocybin/. Accessed October 16, 2012.

Cox, Harvey. 1977. *Turning East: The Promise and Peril of the New Orientalism.* New York: Simon & Schuster.

———. 2009. *The Future of Faith.* New York: HarperCollins.

Cozzi, Nicholas V. 2011. University of Wisconsin. Personal communication.

de Boer, Jelle Z., John R. Hale, and Jeffrey P. Chanton. 2001. "New Evidence for the Geological Origins of the Ancient Delphic Oracle (Greece)." *Geology* 29, no. 8: 707–11.

de Mause, Lloyd, ed. 1975. *The New Psychohistory.* New York: Psychohistory Press.

———. 1982. *Foundations of Psychohistory.* New York: Creative Roots.

de Ropp, Robert S. 1968. *The Master Game: Beyond the Drug Experience.* New York: Delta Books.

"Designer Hens Lay Anti-Cancer Eggs." 2007. Medical News Today. www .medicalnewstoday.com/articles/60816.php. Accessed October 16, 2012.

Devereux, Paul. 1997. *The Long Trip: The Prehistory of Psychedelia.* New York: Penguin.

Doblin, Richard. 1991. "Pahnke's 'Good Friday Experiment': A Long-term Follow-up and Methodological Critique." *Journal of Transpersonal Psychology* 23: 1–28.

———. 2001. "Pahnke's Good Friday Experiment: A Long-term Follow-up and Methodological Critique." Chapter 7 in *Psychoactive Sacramentals: Essays on Entheogens and Religion,* edited by Thomas B. Roberts. San Francisco: Council on Spiritual Practices.

Dyck, Erica. 2008. *Psychedelic Psychiatry: LSD from Clinic to Campus.* Baltimore, Md.: The Johns Hopkins University Press.

Egan, Kieran. 1997. *The Educated Mind: How Cognitive Tools Shape Our Understanding.* Chicago: University of Chicago Press.

Eliade, Mircea. 1972. *Shamanism: Archaic Techniques of Ecstasy.* (Bollingen Series). Princeton: Princeton University Press.

Engelbart, Douglas C. 1962. *Augmenting Human Intellect: A Conceptual Framework.* Summary Report AFOSR-3233. Menlo Park, Calif.: Stanford Research Institute.

Fadiman, James. 1965. Behavior Change Following Psychedelic (LSD) Therapy. Unpublished doctoral dissertation for Stanford University, Stanford, Calif.

———. 2011. *The Psychedelic Explorer's Guide: Safe, Therapeutic, and Sacred Journeys.* Rochester, Vt.: Park Street Press.

Fisher, G. 1970. "Psychotherapy for the Dying: Principles and Illustrative Cases with Special Reference to the Use of LSD." *OMEGA* 1: 3–15.

Forman, Robert K., ed. 1997. *The Problem of Pure Consciousness: Mysticism and Philosophy.* New York: Oxford University Press.

Frances, Sherana Harriet. 2001. *Drawing It Out: Befriending the Unconscious.* Sarasota, Fl.: Multidisciplinary Association for Psychedelic Studies.

Freeman, Lyn. 2009. "Effects of Imagery on Physiology and Biochemistry." In *Mosby's Complementary & Alternative Medicine: A Research-Based Approach.* St. Louis, Mo.: Elsevier (Third Edition).

"Functioning Synapse Created Using Carbon Nanotubes: Devices Might be Used in Brain Prostheses or Synthetic Brains." 2011. www.sciencedaily.com/releases/2011/04/110421151921.htm. Accessed October 17, 2012.

Gardner, Howard. 1983. *Frames of Mind: The Theory of Multiple Intelligences.* New York: Basic Books.

Gilmour, David, Bob Ezrin, and Roger Waters (Directors). 1979. *Pink Floyd: The Wall.* Berre les Alpes, France: Super Bear Studios.

Glock, Martha H., Patricia A. Heller, and Daniel Malamud. 1992. *Saliva as Diagnostic Fluid: January 1982 through April 1992.* Bethesda, Md.: National Library of Medicine, National Institutes of Health.

"Glowing Cats Shed Light on AIDS." 2011. BBC News, Science & Environment. www.bbc.co.uk/news/science-environment-14882008. Accessed October 16, 2012.

Goldsmith, Neal M. 2011. *Psychedelic Healing: The Promise of Entheogens for Psychotherapy and Spiritual Development.* Rochester, Vt.: Healing Arts Press.

Greely, Henry. 2009. "Brain Boosters: How Should We Deal with Cognitive-enhancing Drugs?" *Stanford Magazine,* March/April. www.stanfordalumni .org/news/magazine/2009/marapr/farm/news/greely.html. Accessed Mar. 24, 2009.

Greely, Henry, B. Sahakian, J. Harris, et al. 2008. "Toward Responsible Use of Cognitive-enhancing Drugs by the Healthy." *Nature* 456, no. 7223: 702–5.

Griffiths, Roland. 2009. "Psilocybin and Experimental Mystical Experience." PowerPoint lecture to TEDxAtlantic. http://tedxmidatlantic.com/2009-video/#RolandGriffiths. Accessed August 26, 2010.

Griffiths, Roland, and Charles Grob. 2010. "Hallucinogens as Medicine." *Scientific American,* Dec.: 76–79.

Griffiths, Roland, William Richards, Una McCann, et al. 2006. "Psilocybin Can Occasion Mystical-type Experiences Having Substantial and Sustained Personal Meaning and Spiritual Significance." *Psychopharmacology* 187, no. 3: 268–83.

———. 2008. "Mystical-type Experiences Occasioned by Psilocybin Mediate the Attribution of Personal Meaning and Spiritual Significance 14 Months Later." *Journal of Psychopharmacology* 6: 621–32.

Griffiths, Roland, Matthew W. Johnson, William A. Richards, et al. 2011. "Psilocybin Occasioned Mystical-type Experiences' Immediate and Persisting Dose-related Effects." *Psychopharmacology* 218: 649–65.

Griffiths et al. Psilocybin Studies at the Johns Hopkins University. http://csp .org/psilocybin/. Accessed August, 25, 2011.

Grinspoon, Lester, and James B. Bakalar. 1979. *Psychedelic Drugs Reconsidered.* New York: Basic Books.

Grob, Charles. 2007. "The Use of Psilocybin in Patients with Advanced Cancer and Existential Anxiety." Chapter 11 in vol. 1 of *Psychedelic Medicine: New Evidence for Hallucinogenic Substances as Treatments,* edited by Michael Winkelman and Thomas B. Roberts. Westport, Conn.: Praeger.

Grob, Charles S., Alicia L. Danforth, Gurpreet S. Chopra, et al. "Pilot Study of Psilocybin Treatment for Anxiety in Patients with Advanced-Stage Cancer." *Archives of General Psychiatry* 68, no. 1: 71–78.

Grof, Stanislav. 1975. *Realms of the Human Unconscious: Observations from LSD Research.* New York: Viking Press.

———. 1977. "The Perinatal Roots of Wars, Revolutions, and Totalitarianism: Observations from LSD Research." *Journal of Psychohistory* 4, no. 3: 269–308.

———. 1980. *LSD Psychotherapy.* Pomona, Calif.: Hunter House.

———. 1985. *Beyond the Brain: Birth, Death and Transcendence in Psychotherapy.* Albany, N.Y.: State University of New York Press.

———. 2001. *LSD Psychotherapy.* Santa Cruz, Calif.: Multidisciplinary Association for Psychedelic Studies.

———. 2006. *The Ultimate Journey: Consciousness and the Mystery of Death.* Santa Cruz, Calif.: Multidisciplinary Association for Psychedelic Studies.

———. 2009. *LSD: Doorway to the Numinous.* Rochester, Vt: Inner Traditions, Bear & Company.

———. 2012. "Revision and Revisioning of Psychology: Legacy from Half a Century of Consciousness Research." www.stanislavgrof.com/pdf/Revision.Revisioning.Psychology_Legacy-9.2012.pdf. Accessed September 21, 2012.

Grof, Stanislav, and Hal Zina Bennett. 1992. *The Holotropic Mind: The Three Levels of Human Consciousness and How They Shape Our Lives.* New York: HarperCollins.

Grof, Stanislav, Louis E. Goodman, William A. Richards, et al. 1973. "LSD-assisted Psychotherapy in Patients with Terminal Cancer." *International Pharmacopsychiatry* 8: 129–44.

Grof, Stanislav, and Christina Grof. 1980. *Beyond Death: The Gates of Consciousness.* New York: Thames and Hudson.

Grof, Stanislav, and Joan Halifax. 1977. *The Human Encounter with Death.* New York: E. P. Dutton.

Groisman, Alberto, and Marlene Dobkin de Rios. 2007. "Ayahuasca, the U.S.

Supreme Court, and the UDV-U.S. Government Case: Culture, Religion, and Implications of a Legal Dispute." Chapter 14 in vol. 1 of *Psychedelic Medicine,* edited by Michael Winkelman and Thomas B. Roberts. Westport, Conn.: Praeger.

Guss, Jeffrey. 2011. Bellevue Hospital–New York University. Personal communication.

"G. W. Pharmaceutical, Cannabis Company GW Pharmaceuticals raises $34.5mm in IPO." 2001. Elsevier Business Intelligence. http://sis.windhover.com/buy/abstract.php?id=200130273. Accessed May 20, 2012.

Hale, John R., Jelle Z. de Boer, Jeffrey Chanton, et al. 2003. "Questioning the Delphic Oracle." *Scientific American.* August: 66–73.

Hall, Donald. 1989. *Dock Ellis in the Country of Baseball.* Fireside Press, Los Angeles.

Harman, Willis, Robert H. McKim, Robert E. Mogar, et al. 1966. "Psychedelic Agents in Creative Problem Solving: A Pilot Study." *Psychological Reports* 19: 211–27.

Harner, Michael, ed. 1973. *Hallucinogens and Shamanism.* Oxford, U.K.: Oxford University Press.

"Harvard Scientists to Make LSD Factory from Microbes." 2011. The Guardian. www.guardian.co.uk/science/blog/2011/jun/21/scientists-make-lsd-from-microbes. Accessed June 6, 2011.

Hayes, Charles. 2000. *Tripping: An Anthology of True-life Psychedelic Adventures.* New York: Penguin Putnam.

Hayes, Rosemary. 1975. "Do You Have Your Dream for English?" in *Four Psychologies Applied to Education: Freudian, Behavioral, Humanistic, Transpersonal,* edited by Thomas B. Roberts. Cambridge, Mass.: Schenkman.

Healy, Melissa. 2011. Turn On, Tune In, Get Better? *The Los Angeles Times.* Nov. 30. Home Edition. http://articles.latimes.com/print/nov/30/health/la-he-drugs-of-abuse-20111130. Accessed October 16, 2012.

Heffter Research Institute. www.heffter.org.

Heifer International. 2011. *The Most Important Gift Catalog in the World.* Little Rock, Ark.: Heifer International.

Heinrich, Clark. 2002. *Magic Mushrooms in Religion and Alchemy.* Rochester, Vt.: Park Street Press.

Henricks, Gay, and Russel Wills. 1977. *The Centering Book: Awareness Activities for Children and Adults to Relax the Body and Mind.* Englewood Cliffs, N.J.: Prentice-Hall.

Hendricks, Gay, and Thomas B. Roberts. 1979. *The Second Centering Book: More Awareness Activities for Children and Adults to Relax the Body and Mind.* Englewood Cliffs, N.J.: Prentice-Hall.

Hentzen, Annelie, and Torsten Passie. 2010. *The Pharmacology of LSD: A Critical Review.* Beckley Foundation and Oxford University Press.

Hillman, D. C. A. 2008. *The Chemical Muse: Drug Use and the Roots of Western Civilization.* New York: St. Martin's Press.

Hoffman, Edward. 1988. *The Right to Be Human: A Biography of Abraham Maslow.* Los Angeles: Jeremy P. Tarcher, Inc.

Hood, Ralph W., Jr. 1975. "Construction and Preliminary Validation of a Measure of Reported Mystical Experience." *Journal for the Scientific Study of Consciousness* 14, no. 1: 29–41.

———. 1995. "The Facilitation of Religious Experience." Chapter 24 in *Handbook of Religious Experience,* edited by Ralph W. Hood Jr. Birmingham, Ala.: Religious Education Press.

———. 2006. "The Common Core Thesis in the Study of Mysticism." Chapter 5 in *Where God and Science Meet,* vol. 3 of *The Psychology of Religious Experience,* edited by Patrick McNamara. Westport, Conn.: Praeger.

Hood, Ralph W., Jr., Ronald J. Morris, and P. J. Watson. 1993. "Further Factor Analysis of Hood's Mysticism Scale." *Psychological Reports* 73, no. 1: 1176–78.

Hood, Ralph W., Jr., Bernard Spilka, Bruce Hunsberger, and Richard Gorsuch. 1996. *The Psychology of Religion: An Empirical Approach.* New York: Guilford Press.

"Horizon: Psychedelic Science." 1997. BBC-TV Program No. 60/LSF/A611A. Broadcast 13 Jan. www.bbc.co.uk/horizon/psychetran.shtml. Accessed October 17, 2012.

"Hublot Chronograph." 2012. How to Spend It. www.howtospendit.com/#!/articles/7009-eclectibles-hublot-watch. Accessed May 13, 2012.

Huxley, Aldous. 1962. *Island.* New York: Harper and Row.

Ikemi, Y., S. Nakagawa, T. Nakagawa, et al. 1975. "Psychosomatic Consideration of Cancer Patients Who Have Made a Narrow Escape from Death." *Dynamiche Psychiatry* 31: 77–92.

Jacobson, B., G. Eklund, L. Hamberger, et al. 1987. "Perinatal Origin of Adult Self-destructive Behavior." *Acta Psychiatrica Scandinavia* 79 (October): 364–71.

Jacobson, B., and Marc Bygdeman. 1998. "Obstetric Care and Proneness of Offspring to Suicide as Adults: Case-Control Study." *British Medical Journal* 317: 1,346ff.

James, William. 1958. "Lectures XVI and XVII, Mysticism." In *The Varieties of Religious Experience: A Study in Human Nature, Being the Gifford Lectures on Natural Religion Delivered at Edinburgh in 1901–1902*. New York: Mentor Edition, New American Library.

Jemmott, J. B., and K. Magloire. 1988. "Academic Stress, Social Support, and Secretory Immunoglobulin A." *Journal of Personality and Social Psychology* 55: 803–10.

Jesse, Robert. 2012. "About the Council on Spiritual Practices: Code of Ethics for Spiritual Guides." In *Spiritual Growth with Entheogens: Psychoactive Sacramentals and Human Transformation*, edited by Thomas B. Roberts. Rochester, Vt.: Park Street Press.

Johnson, Ken. 2011. *Are You Experienced? How Psychedelic Consciousness Transformed Modern Art*. Munich/London/New York: Prestel.

Johnson, Matthew W., William A. Richards, and Roland R. Griffiths. 2008. "Human Hallucinogen Research: Guidelines for Safety." *Journal of Psychopharmacology* 22, no. 6: 603–20.

Kackar, Hayal, and Thomas B. Roberts. 2005. "*Fight Club* and the Basic Perinatal Matrices: A Movie Analysis via a Grofian Frame." *Journal of Transpersonal Psychology* 37, no. 1: 44–51.

Kapleau, Philip. 1965. *The Three Pillars of Zen*. Boston: Beacon Press.

Kast, Eric C. 1966. "Pain and LSD-25: A Theory of Attenuation of Anticipation." Chapter 14 in *LSD: The Consciousness-expanding Drug,* edited by D. Solomon. New York: G. P. Putnam's.

Katz, Stephen, ed. 1983. *Mysticism and Religious Traditions*. Oxford, U.K.: Oxford University Press.

Kleiman, Mark. 2011. "Mysticism in the Lab." www.samefacts.com/2011/06/drug-policy/mysticism-in-the-lab/. Accessed June 17, 2011.

Kubie, Lawrence S. 1954. "The Forgotten Man of Education." *Harvard Alumni Bulletin* 56: 349–53.

Kuhn, Thomas S. 1962. *The Structure of Scientific Revolutions*. Chicago: University of Chicago Press.

Kung, Hans, Josef Ess, Heinrich von Stietencron, and Heinz Bechert. 1986. *Christianity and the World Religions: Paths to Dialogue with Islam, Hinduism and Buddhism*. Garden City, N.Y.: Doubleday.

Labate, Beatriz Caiuby. 2011. "Paradoxes of Ayahuasca Expansion: The UDV-DEA Agreement and the Limits of Freedom of Religion." *Drugs: Education, Prevention and Policy*. doi: 10.3109/09687637.2011.606397. Accessed Nov. 3, 2011.

Lambert, R. B., and N. K. Lambert. 1995. "The Effects of Humor on Secretory Immunoglobulin A Levels in School-aged Children." *Pediatric Nursing* 21, no. 1 (Jan-Feb): 16–19, 28–29.

Lee, Martin A., and Bruce Shlain. 1994. *Acid Dreams: The Complete Social History of LSD: The CIA, the Sixties, and Beyond*. New York: Grove Press.

Lerner, Michael, and Michael Lyvers. 2006. "Values and Beliefs of Psychedelic Drug Users: A Cross-cultural Study." *Journal of Psychoactive Drugs* 38, no. 2 (June): 143–47.

"LSD Studies with Autistic Children" www.neurodiversity.com/lsd/html. Accessed Aug. 11, 2011.

MacLean, Katherine A., Matthew W. Johnson, and Roland R. Griffiths. 2011. "Mystical Experiences Occasioned by the Hallucinogen Psilocybin Lead to Increases in the Personality Domain of Openness." *Journal of Psychopharmacology* 25, no 11: 1453–61.

Markoff, John. 2006. *What the Dormouse Said: How the Sixties Counterculture Shaped the Personal Computer Industry*. New York: Penguin.

Maslow, Abraham H. 1954. *Motivation and Personality*. New York: Harper and Row.

———. 1962. *Toward a Psychology of Being*. Princeton, N.J.: Van Nostrand.

———. 1964. *Religions, Values, and Peak Experiences*. New York: Penguin Books.

———. 1969. "Theory Z." *Journal of Transpersonal Psychology* 1, no. 2: 31–47.

———. 1971. "Various Meanings of Transcendence" and "A Theory of Metamotivation: The Biological Rooting of the Value-Life." Chapters 21 and 23 in *The Farther Reaches of Human Nature.* New York: Viking Press.

Masters, Robert E. L., and Jean Houston. 1968. *Psychedelic Art.* New York: Grove Press.

Matossian, Mary K. 1989. *Poisons of the Past: Molds, Epidemics, and History.* New Haven: Yale University Press.

Matsunaga, Masahiro, Tokiko Isowa, Kenta Kimura, et al. 2008. "Associations among Central Nervous, Endocrine, and Immune Activities when Positive Emotions Are Elicited by Looking at a Favorite Person." *Brain, Behavior, and Immunity* 22, no. 3 (March): 408–17.

McCoubrie, R. C., and A. N. Davies. 2006. "Is There a Correlation between Spirituality and Anxiety and Depression in Patients with Advanced Cancer?" *Support Care Cancer* 14: 379–85.

McKenna, Dennis. 2011. University of Minnesota. Personal communication.

McLean, Cory Y., Philip L. Reno, Alex A. Pollen, et al. 2011. "Human-specific Loss of Regulatory DNA and the Evolution of Human-specific Traits." *Nature* 471: 216–19.

Meares, A. 1979. "Regression of Cancer of the Rectum after Intensive Meditation." *Medical Journal of Australia* 2 (Nov.17): 539–40.

Medline. 1993–2011. National Library of Medicine. www.nlm.nih.gov.

Merlin, Mark D. 2003. "Archeological Evidence for the Tradition of Psychoactive Plant Use in the Old World." *Economic Botany* 57, no. 3: 295–323.

Metzner, Ralph. 2002. "Ritual Approaches to Working with Sacred Medicine Plants." Chapter 15 in *Hallucinogens, A Reader,* edited by Charles Grob. New York: Tarcher/Putnam.

Miller, William R., and Janet C'de Baca. 2001. *Quantum Change: When Epiphanies and Sudden Insights Transform Ordinary Lives.* New York: Guilford Press.

———. 2005. "Anatomy of a Quantum Change." *Spirituality & Health*, February.

Mithoefer, Michael. 2007. "MDMA-assisted Psychotherapy for the Treatment of Post-traumatic Stress Disorder." In Vol. 1 of Michael Winkelman and Thomas B. Roberts, eds. *Psychedelic Medicine: New Evidence for Hallucinogenic Substances as Treatments.* Westport, Conn.: Praeger.

Mithoefer, Michael C., M. Y. Wagner, A. T. Mithoefer, et al. 2011. "The Safety and Efficacy of {+/-}3,4-methylenedioxymethamphetamine-assisted Psychotherapy in Subjects with Chronic, Treatment-resistant Posttraumatic Stress Disorder: The First Randomized Controlled Pilot Study." *Psychopharmacology* 25, no. 4: 439–52.

Mogar, Robert E., and Robert W. Aldrich. 1969. "The Use of Psychedelic Agents with Autistic Schizophrenic Children." *Psychedelic Review* 10: 5–13.

Mojeilko, Valerie. 2010. "MAPS Attends American Psychological Association Conference." *MAPS Bulletin* XX, no. 3.

Morris, Kelly. 2006. "Hallucinogen Research Inspires Neurotheology." *The Lancet Neurology* 5, no. 9 (Sept): 732.

———. 2008. "Research on Psychedelics Moves into the Mainstream." *The Lancet* 371: 1,491–92.

Mullis, Kary. 1998. *Dancing Naked in the Mind Field*. New York: Pantheon Press.

Nerurkar, A., G. Yeh, R. B. Davis, et al. 2011. "When Conventional Medical Providers Recommend Unconventional Medicine: Results of a National Study." *Archives of Internal Medicine* 171, no. 9: 862–64.

"New Hope for Children with Craniosynostosis: Developing Technologies to Improve the Treatment for Premature Fusion of Skull Bones in Children." 2011. *ScienceDaily*. www.sciencedaily.com/releases/2011/09/110906152455 .htm. Accessed September 19, 2011.

Nichols, David, and Benjamin R. Chemel. 2006. "The Neuropharmacology of Religious Experience: Hallucinogens and the Experience of the Divine." Chapter 1 in *Where God and Science Meet: How Brain and Evolutionary Studies Alter Our Understanding of Religion*. Vol. 3 of *The Psychology of Religious Experience*, edited by Patrick McNamara. Westport, Conn.: Praeger.

Novotney, Amy. 2010. "Research on Psychedelics Makes a Comeback." *American Psychological Association Monitor*, Nov.

O'Regan, Brendon, and Caryle Hirshberg. 1993. *Spontaneous Remission: An Annotated Bibliography*. Sausalito, Calif.: Institute of Noetic Sciences.

Pahnke, W.N. 1969. "The Psychedelic Mystical Experience in the Human Encounter with Death." *Harvard Theological Review* 62: 1–21.

Pahnke, Walter N., and William A. Richards. 1966. "Implications of LSD and Experimental Mysticism." *Journal of Religion and Health* 5, no. 3: 175–208.

Parker, Alan, Director. 1982. *Pink Floyd: The Wall*. New York: MGM/UA.

"'Pass It On' The Story of Bill Wilson and How the A.A. Message Reached the World." 1984. New York: Alcoholics Anonymous World Services.

Passie, Torsten. 1997. *Psycholytic and Psychedelic Therapy Research 1931–1995: A Complete International Bibliography*. Hannover, Germany: Laurentis Publishers.

Perrine, Daniel. 1996. "Chemical/Substance/Drug Addiction/Dependence/ Abuse." In *The Chemistry of Mind-Altering Drugs: History, Pharmacology, and Cultural Context*. Washington, D.C.: American Chemical Society.

Persisting Effects Questionnaire. 2012. "Electronic Supplementary Material, Table 2, Altruism Scale." www.springerlink.com/content/ v2175688r1w4862x/213_2006_Article_457_ESM.html. Accessed May 13, 2012.

Philipkoski, Kristen. 2002. "RIP: Alba, the Glowing Bunny." Wired. www .wired.com/medtech/health/news/2002/08/54399?currentPage=all. Accessed October 16, 2012.

Piccardi, Luigi, Cassandra Monti, Orlando Vaselli, et al. 2008. "Scent of a Myth: Tectonics, Geochemistry and Geomythology at Delphi (Greece)." *Journal of the Geological Society* 165, no. 1: 1–5.

Rees, Alan. 2004. "Nobel Prize Genius Crick Was High on LSD When He Discovered the Secret of Life." *Mail on Sunday* (London), August 8. Section FB: 44–45.

"Repeated Stress in Pregnancy Linked to Children's Behavior." 2011. *Science Daily*. www.sciencedaily.com/releases/2011/04/110420111900.htm. Accessed October 16, 2012.

Rhead, John C. 1977. "The Use of Psychedelic Drugs in the Treatment of Severely Disturbed Children: A Review." *Journal of Psychedelic Drugs* 9, no. 2: 95–101.

Richards, William A. 1978. *Peak Experiences, Counseling, and the Human Encounter with Death: An Empirical Study of the Efficacy of DPT-assisted Counseling in Enhancing the Quality of Life of Persons with Terminal Cancer and Their Closest Family Members*. Washington, D.C.: Catholic University of America.

Richards, William, John Rhead, Franco DiLeo, et al. 1977. "The Peak Experience Variable in DPT-assisted Psychotherapy with Cancer Patients." *Journal of Psychedelic Drugs* 9, no. 1: 1–10.

Riedlinger, Thomas J. 1982. "Sartre's Rite of Passage." *Journal of Transpersonal Psychology* 14, no. 2: 105–23.

———. ed. 1990. *The Sacred Mushroom Seeker: Essays for R. Gordon Wasson.* Portland, Ore.: Dioscorides Press.

Riedlinger, Thomas J., and June Riedlinger. 1986. "Taking Birth Trauma Seriously." *Medical Hypotheses* 19: 15–25.

Roberts, Andy. 2008. *Albion Dreaming: A Popular History of LSD in Britain.* London: Marshall Cavendish.

Roberts, Thomas B. 1978. "Beyond Self-Actualization." *ReVision* 1, no. 1 (Winter): 42–46.

———. 1986. "*Brainstorm*: A Psychological Odyssey." *Journal of Humanistic Psychology* 26, no. 1 (Winter): 126–36.

———. 1989. "Multistate Education: Metacognitive Implications of the Mindbody Psychotechnologies." *Journal of Transpersonal Psychology* 21, no. 1: 83–102.

———. 1998. "Multidisciplinary Approaches to Psychedelic Scholarship (MAPS)." *Newsletter of the Multidisciplinary Association for Psychedelic Studies, MAPS* 8, no. 1 (Spring): 38–41. Available online at niu.academia .edu/ThomasRoberts and www.maps.org/news-letters/v08n1/08138rob .html.

———. 2006. *Psychedelic Horizons: Snow White, Immune System, Multistate Mind, Enlarging Education.* Exeter, U.K.: Imprint Academic.

———. ed. 2012. *Spiritual Growth with Entheogens: Psychoactive Sacramentals and Human Transformation.* Rochester, Vt.: Park Street Press.

———. 2012. "Positive Psychology: The Science of Happiness and Flourishing." Academia.edu. www.academia.edu/1443561/Book_review_Positive_ Psychology_The_Science_of_Happiness_and_Flourishing. Accessed October 16, 2012.

———. Foundations of Psychedelic Studies. www.niu.academia.edu/Thomas Roberts.

———. 2010. Foundations of Psychedelic Studies. http://niu.academia.edu/ ThomasRoberts/Talks/18125/Foundations_of_Psychedelic_Studies_

PowerPoint_slides. Lecture at *Psychedelic Science in the Twenty-first Century*, San Jose, Calif. April 2010.

Roberts, Thomas B., and Paula Jo Hruby. 1995–2001. "Religion and Psychoactive Sacraments: An Entheogen Chrestomathy." www.csp.org/chrestomathy. Accessed May 31, 2011.

Roberts, Thomas B., and Bruce Sewick. 2010. "University Courses on Psychedelics in Higher Education." www.maps.org/videos/source4/video13.html. Accessed October 16, 2012.

Roberts, Thomas B., and Michael Winkelman. 2013. "Psychedelic Induced Transpersonal Experiences, Therapies, and Their Implications for Transpersonal Psychology." In *Handbook of Transpersonal Psychology,* edited by Harris Friedman and Glenn Hartelius. Hoboken, N.J.: Wiley-Blackwell.

Robinson, Monique, Eugen Mattes, Wendy Oddy, et al. 2011. "Prenatal Stress and Risk of Behavioral Morbidity from Age 2 to 14 Years: The Influence of the Number, Type, and Timing of Stressful Life Events." *Development and Psychopathology* 23, no. 2: 155–68.

Ross, Stephen, et al. 2012. NYU Program in Psychedelic Psychotherapy. Fall 2012–Spring 2013 Syllabus. Bellevue Hospital, New York.

Ross, Stephen, et al. 2012. "Psilocybin Advanced Cancer Anxiety Study." ClinicalTrials.gov. http://clinicaltrials.gov/ct2/show/NCT00957359. Accessed October 16, 2012.

Rousseau, P. 2000. "Spirituality and the Dying Patient." *Journal of Clinical Oncology* 18: 2000–2002.

Ruck, Carl A. P., Blaise Staples, and Clark Heinrich. 2001. *The Apples of Apollo: Pagan and Christian Mysteries of the Eucharist*. Durham, N.C.: Carolina Academic Press.

Rudgley, Richard. 1993. *Essential Substances in Society: A Cultural History of Intoxicants in Society*. New York: Kodansha International.

———. 1999. *The Lost Civilizations of the Stone Age*. New York: The Free Press.

Sacramento Bee. 2012. "Software Pioneer Leaves $10 Million Bequest to Five Leading Non-profits in Health and Drug Policy Reform." Multidisciplinary Association for Psychedelic Studies (MAPS). www.sacbee.com/2012/05/30/4526574/software-pioneer-leaves-10-million.html#storylink=cpy. Accessed June 1, 2012.

Samorini, Giorgio. 2000. *Animals and Psychedelics: The Natural World and the Instinct to Alter Consciousness*. Rochester, Vt.: Park Street Press.

Schachter-Shalomi, Zalman. 2005. "Transcending Religious Boundaries." In *Higher Wisdom: Eminent Elders Explore the Continuing Impact of Psychedelics*, edited by Roger Walsh and Charles Grob. Albany, New York: SUNY Press.

Schilder, Johannes N. 2011. Personal communication.

Schilder, Johannes N., Marco J. de Vries, Karl Goodkin, et al. 2004. "Psychological Changes Preceding Spontaneous Remission of Cancer." *Clinical Case Studies* 3, no. 4: 288–312.

Schultes, Richard, and Albert Hofmann. 1992. *Plants of the Gods: Their Sacred, Healing and Hallucinogenic Powers*. Rochester, Vt.: Healing Arts Press.

Schwartz, Jeffrey M., and Sharon Begley. 2003. *The Mind and the Brain: Neuroplasticity and the Power of Mental Force*. New York: Harper Perennial.

Seaman, Gary, and Jane S. Day, eds. 1994. *Ancient Traditions: Shamanism in Central Asia and the Americas*. Niwot, Colo.: University Press of Colorado and Denver Museum of Natural History.

Sessa, Ben. 2012. *The Psychedelic Renaissance: Reassessing the Role of Psychedelic Drugs in 21st Century Psychiatry and Society*. London: Muswell Hill Press.

Shanon, Benny. 2002. *The Antipodes of the Mind: Charting the Phenomenology of the Ayahuasca Experience*. Oxford, U.K.: Oxford University Press.

Shulgin, Alexander, Tania Manning, and Paul F. Daley. 2011. *The Shulgin Index: Psychedelic Phenethylamines and Related Compounds*. Berkeley, Calif.: Transform Press.

Shulgin, Alexander, and Wendy Perry. 2002. *The Simple Plant Isoquinolines*. Berkeley, Calif.: Transform Press.

Shulgin, Alexander, and Ann Shulgin. 1991. *PiHKAL: A Chemical Love Story*. Berkeley, Calif.: Transform Press.

———. 1997. *TiHKAL: The Continuation*. Berkeley, Calif.: Transform Press.

Siegel, Ronald K. 1989. *Intoxication: Life in Pursuit of Artificial Paradise*. New York: E. P Dutton.

"Single Dose of 'Magic Mushrooms' Hallucinogen May Create Lasting Personality Change, Study Suggests." 2011. *Science Daily*. www.sciencedaily.com/releases/2011/09/110929074205.htm. Accessed Retrieved May 12, 2012.

Slater, Lauren. 2012. "Is the World Ready for Medical Hallucinogens?—A

Kaleidoscope at the End of the Tunnel." *The New York Times Magazine,* April 22: 56–60, 66.

Smile Train. 2011. Washington, D.C. www.SmileTrain.org.

Smith, Huston. 1964. "Do Drugs Have Religious Import?" *The Journal of Philosophy* LXI: 517–30.

———. 1977. *Forgotten Truth: The Primordial Tradition.* New York: Harper & Row.

———. 2000. *Cleansing the Doors of Perception: The Religious Significance of Entheogenic Plants and Chemicals.* New York: Tarcher/Putnam.

———. 2008. *The World's Religions.* New York: HarperCollins.

Smith, Huston, and Ruben Snake. 1996. *One Nation Under God: The Triumph of the Native American Church.* Santa Fe, N.Mex.: City Light Publishers.

Snyder, Allan. 2009. "Explaining and Inducing Savant Skills: Privileged Access to Lower Level, Less-processed Information." *Philosophical Transactions of the Royal Society B: Biological Sciences* 364: 1,399–1,405.

Society for the Anthropology of Consciousness. www.sacaaa.org/SAC.

Spiller, Henry A., John R. Hale, and Jelle Z. de Boer. 2002. "The Delphic Oracle: A Multidisciplinary Defense of the Gaseous Vent Theory." *Journal of Clinical Toxicology* 40, no. 2: 89–196.

Stace, Walter T. 1961. *Mysticism and Philosophy.* London: Macmillan.

Steenhuysen, Julie. 2011. "How Humans Got Big Brains, Barbless Penises." Reuters.com. www.reuters.com/article/2011/03/09/us-humans-dna-idUSTRE7285MF20110309. Accessed December 5, 2012.

Sternberg, Robert J. 1988. *The Triarchic Mind: A New Theory of Human Intelligence.* New York: Penguin.

Stevens, Jay. 1987. *Storming Heaven: LSD and the American Dream.* New York: Harper & Row.

Stockler, M. R., R. O'Connell, R. K. Nowak, et al. 2007. "Effects of Sertraline on Symptoms and Survival in Patients with Advanced Cancer, but without Major Depression: A Placebo-controlled Double-blind Randomized Trial." *Lancet Oncology* 8: 603–12.

Stolaroff, Myron. 1994. "MDMA Plus LSD." In *Thanatos to Eros: Thirty-five Years of Psychedelic Exploration.* Berlin: VWB–Verlag fur Wissenschaft und Bildung.

———. 2004. *The Secret Chief Revealed: Conversations with a Pioneer of the Underground Psychedelic Therapy Movement.* Multidisciplinary Association for Psychedelic Studies, Sarasota, Fl. (now Santa Cruz, Calif.)

———. 2012. "A Protocol for a Sacramental Service." Chapter 16 in *Spiritual Growth with Entheogens*, Thomas B. Roberts, ed. Rochester, Vt.: Inner Traditions.

Stone, Arthur A., Christine A. Macro, Charles E. Cruise, et al. 1996. "Are Stress-induced Immunological Changes Mediated by Mood? A Closer Look at How Both Desirable and Undesirable Daily Events Influence sIgA Antibody." *International Journal of Behavioral Medicine* 3: 1–13.

Stone, Arthur A., John M. Neale, Donald S. Cox, et al. 1994. "Daily Events Are Associated with a Secretory Immune Response to an Oral Antigen in Men." *Health Psychology* 13, no. 5: 440–46.

Stone, Arthur A., Heiddis Valdimarsdottir, Lina Jandorf, et al. 1987. "Evidence that Secretory IgA Antibody Is Associated with Daily Mood." *Journal of Personality and Social Psychology* 25, no. 5: 988–93.

Substance Abuse and Mental Health Services Administration. 2010. "Table 1.1A. Types of Illicit Drug Use in Lifetime, Past Year, and Past Month among Persons Aged 12 or Older: Numbers in Thousands, 2008 and 2009." In *Results from the 2009 National Survey on Drug Use and Health: Detailed Tables* (Office of Applied Studies, NSDUH Series H-38A, HHS Publication No. SMA 10-4856Findings). Rockville, Md.

Talbot, Margaret. 2009. "Brain Gain: The Underground World of 'Neuroenhancing' Drugs." *The New Yorker,* April 27: 32–43.

Tart, Charles T., ed. 1969. *Altered States of Consciousness: A Book of Readings.* New York: John Wiley and Sons.

———. 1991. Influence of Previous Psychedelic Drug Experience on Students of Tibetan Buddhism: A Preliminary Exploration. *Journal of Transpersonal Psychology* 23, no. 2: 139–74.

———. 2001. *Mind Science.* Novato, Calif.: Wisdom Editions.

Treffert, Darold. 2011. "Extraordinary People: The Savant Syndrome." www.btci.org/bioethics/2011/videos2011/default.html. Accessed June 19, 2011.

Trumbull, Douglas, producer and director. 1983. *Brainstorm.* New York: MGM/UA.

Tupper, Kenneth W. 2003. "Entheogens & Education: Exploring the Potential of Psychoactives as Educational Tools." *Journal of Drug Education and Awareness* 1, no. 2: 145–61.

———. 2011. *Ayahuasca, Entheogenic Education & Public Policy.* Unpublished doctoral dissertation, University of British Columbia, Vancouver, BC.

U.S. National Institutes of Health. www.clinicaltrials.gov.

Valdimarsdottir, Heiddis B., and Dana H. Bovbjerg. 1997. "Positive and Negative Mood: Association with Natural Killer Cell Activity." *Psychology and Health* 12: 319–27.

Valdimarsdottir, Heiddis B., and Arthur A. Stone. 1997. "Psychosocial Factors and Secretory Immunoglobulin A." *Critical Reviews in Oral Biology and Medicine* 8, no. 4: 461–74.

Van Dusen, Wilson. 1961. "LSD and the Enlightenment of Zen." *Psychologia* 4: 11–16.

Vaughan, Frances. 1983. "Perception and Knowledge, Reflections on Psychological and Spiritual Learning in the Psychedelic Experience." Chapter 9 in *Psychedelic Reflections,* Lester Grinspoon and James Bakalar. New York: Human Sciences Press.

———. 1987. "A Question of Balance: Health and Pathology in New Religious Movements." In *Spiritual Choices: The Problem of Recognizing Authentic Paths to Inner Transformation,* edited by Dick Anthony, Bruce Ecker, and Ken Wilber. New York: Paragon House. Retrieved from http://csp.org/communities/docs/vaughan-balance.html.

Wainwright, William J. 1981. *Mysticism: A Study of its Nature, Cognitive Value and Moral Implications.* University of Wisconsin Press.

Walsh, Roger. 1982. "Psychedelics and Psychological Well-being." *Journal of Humanistic Psychology* 22: 22–32.

———. 1983. "Psychedelics and Self-actualization." Chapter 10 in *Psychedelic Reflections,* edited by Lester Grinspoon and James B. Bakalar. New York: Human Sciences Press.

———. 2003. Entheogens: True or False? *International Journal of Transpersonal Psychology* 22: 1–6.

———. 2007. *The World of Shamanism.* Woodbury, Minn.: Llewellyn Press.

Walsh, Roger, and Charles Grob, eds. 2005. *Higher Wisdom: Eminent Elders Explore the Continuing Impact of Psychedelics*. Albany, N.Y.: State University of New York Press.

Walsh, Roger, and Frances Vaughan, eds. 1993. *Paths Beyond Ego: The Transpersonal Vision*. New York: Tarcher/Putnam.

Waters, Roger, lyricist. 1979. "In the Flesh?" *Pink Floyd: The Wall*. www .pink-floyd-lyrics.com/html/in-the-flesh-wall-lyrics.html. Accessed April 18, 2011.

Weinstock, C. 1983. "Psychosomatic Elements in 18 Consecutive Cancer Regressions Positively Not Due to Somatic Therapy." *American Society of Psychosomatic Dentistry and Medicine Journal* 30, no. 4: 151–55.

Wilber, Ken. 2000. *Integral Psychology: Consciousness, Spirit, Psychology, Therapy*. Boston, Mass.: Shambhala.

Wilson, Edward O. 1998. *Consilience: The Unity of Knowledge*. New York: Alfred Knopf.

Winkelman, Michael, and Thomas B. Roberts, eds. 2007. *Psychedelic Medicine: New Evidence for Hallucinogenic Substances as Treatments*. 2 vols. Westport, Conn.: Praeger.

Witz, Billy. 2010. "For Ellis, a Long, Strange Trip to a No-Hitter." New York Times online. www.nytimes.com/2010/09/05/sports/baseball/05nohitter .html?_r=0. Accessed October 16, 2012.

Wulff, David. 1991. *Psychology of Religion: Classic and Contemporary Views*. New York: John Wiley.

Zweig, Jason. 2007. *Your Money and Your Brain: How the New Science of Neuroeconomics Can Help Make You Rich*. New York: Simon & Schuster.

Index

Acid Dreams, 152
addiction, 29, 39–40
Against Excess, 58
Albion Dreaming, 152
Alfandre, David, 93
Altered States, 177
Altering Consciousness, 123, 129
altruism, 48–51
Ancient Traditions, 147
Animals and Psychedelics, 156–57
anthropology, 146–49
Antipodes of the Mind, The, 67, 143–44, 148, 214–16, 225
Apples of Apollo, The, 150
archaeology, 149–50
Archives of Internal Medicine, 93
Armstrong, Karen, 56
Ascent of Man, The, 2
athletic feat, on LSD, 157–58
attitude and behavior, changes in, 28–29
Avatar, 176–77
ayahuasca, 67, 77, 130, 143–44, 213, 215

Badiner, Allan, 142
Bakalar, James, 5, 62, 100–101, 148–49, 223

Basic Perinatal Memories (BPMs), 164–65
Bechert, Heinz, 62–63
behavioral psychology, 212
Bejerano, Gill, 187
Bennett, Hal Zina, 47–48
Beyer, Stephan, 228
Beyond Death, 172
Beyond the Brain, 51
birth, 31–32, 163–64. *See also* perinatal level
Bourguignon, Erica, 148
brain, 33, 178–80, 183–88
Brainstorm, 171–72, 177
Bronowski, Jacob, 2
Burnham, Sophie, 68
Bygdeman, Marc, 163

Campbell, Joseph, 173
cancer, 89, 90–91, 99, 103, 108–16
Caporael, Linnda, 154
Cardena, Etzel, 123, 129
Case for God, 56
C'de Baca, Janet, 15–17, 31, 35, 36, 45, 46, 52, 53
Center Book, The, 212

central multistate question, 128, 208, 214

Chemel, Benjamin, 142

Chemical Muse, The, 151

Christianity and the World Religions, 62–63

Christmas Tale, A (Dickens), 15–16

Chronicle of Higher Education, The, 8

Cleansing the Doors of Perception, 60, 68

COEX system, 160–61. *See also* perinatal level

"Cognition of Being in the Peak Experience," 33

cognitive enhancement, psychedelic
    cognitive aspects of psychedelic psychotherapy, 140
    designing and inventing processes, 132–33
    experimental religious studies, 139–40
    experimental studies of abstract concepts, 138–39
    omitted evidence, 144–45
    problem solving, 135–37

cognitive psychology, 212, 215

cognitive studies, 127, 141–45, 217

Cohen, Sidney, 102, 105–6

College DuPage, 228, 229

"Common Core Thesis in the Study of Mysticism, The," 140

Complementary and Alternative Medicine, 92

Compton, William, 12

computer industry, 137–38

concepts, abstract, 138–39

consciousness, 112, 122, 124–25, 147–49

consilience, 142–43

consumption-addicted society, 43–44

conversion, religious, 66–69

Cotton, Ian, 67

Council on Spiritual Practices, 9, 11

Cox, Harvey, 59

Cozzi, Nicholas, 227–28, 229–30

craniosynostosis, 186–87

creation religion/creationists, 27

crowdfunding, hypothetical dialogue, 193–206
    corporations, 204–5
    due diligence, 200–202
    initial public offering (IPO), 199
    making money, 197–98, 200
    publicity, 205–6
    reasons for investing, 195–97
    significant milestones, 202–3
    stockholders, 203–4

Danforth, Alicia, 6, 102, 140

Day, Jane, 147

death, 6, 21, 30, 88–89. *See also* near the end of life

Delphic Oracle, 153

de Mause, Lloyd, 166

de Ropp, Robert S., 40–41

design awards, 230–31

Devereux, Paul, 149–50

Dickens, Charles, 15–16

Doblin, Richard, 74, 139–40

dreams, 210–11

drug-induced mystical experiences
    arguments against, 81–83
    conclusion, 87
    history of, 80–81
    long-term effects of, 83, 85–87
    theoretical framework, 83–85
    See also psychedelic-induced mystical experiences

Drugs and Drug Policies, 58

Dyck, Erica, 152

Economist, The, 8, 10
Ecstasy (MDMA), 71, 107–8, 140,
    181, 226–27
Ecstatic Journey, 68
education
    central multistate question, 208, 214
    development of cognition, 213–14
    higher, 11–12, 216–18
    humanistic, 212–13
    inventing paradigms, 214–16
    multistate capacities, 207–8
    psychotechnologies for, 208–11
    revisioning, 208
    See also Foundations of Psychedelic
        Studies course
ego death/ego loss, 30, 51. *See also*
    transcendence
ego inflation, 76
Eliade, Mircea, 147
Ellis, Dock, 157–58
empirical findings, judging, 129–30
entheogens
    beliefs and knowledge, 65–69
    described, 58, 60
    ethics, 76
    organizations, 77–78
    ritual, 69–76
"Entheogens: True or False?" 80
ergot poisoning, 154
Ess, Josef, 62–63
Essential Substances in Society, 150
ethics, 76
experience-based religion, 55, 57–62

"Facilitation of Religious Experience,
    The," 140

Fadiman, James, 38, 50–51, 72, 76,
    137, 158, 181
Fight Club, 170–71
Forgotten Truth, 84
Forman, Robert, 84
Foundations of Psychedelic Studies
    course
    class discussions, 224
    don't ask, don't tell, 227–28
    guest speakers, 227–28
    hidden allies, 223–24
    higher higher education and,
        228–30
    hints to professors, 221–24
    Internet field trips, 225
    online courses, 217
    overview, 192, 231
    self-selected books, 225
    syllabus, online, 224
    why not to put LSD in friend's
        coffee, 226–27
Frances, Sherana Harriette, 85
Freeman, Lyn, 92
Future of Faith, 59–60

Gardner, Howard, 141
genetic engineering, 182–83
geology, 153
gluttony, 41, 43
Good Friday experiment, 73–75, 78,
    83, 85, 139–40
Gorsuch, Richard, 34
Griffiths, Roland
    "Hallucinogens as Medicine," 10
    "Mystical-type Experiences
        Occasioned by Psilocybin," 16–17,
        58, 75
    on openness, 51

"Psilocybin Can Occasion Mystical-type Experiences," 75

Psilocybin Studies at the Johns Hopkins University in 2011, 78

Grinspoon, Lester, 5, 62, 100–101, 148–49, 223

Grob, Charles, 6, 10, 70, 102, 140, 142, 159

Grof, Christina, 172

Grof, Stanislav
  Beyond Death, 172
  Beyond the Brain, 51
  COEX system, 160–61
  Holotropic Mind, The, 47–48
  Human Encounter with Death, The, 106
  LSD: Doorway to the Numinous, 31, 66–67, 226
  on LSD psychotherapy, 57
  map of the human mind, 31, 126, 127, 159–61
  "Perinatal Roots of Wars, Revolutions, and Totalitarianism, The," 165–66
  psychedelic psychotherapy of, 2
  on psychedelics and spiritual experiences, 49, 81
  Realms of the Human Unconscious, 173
  Ultimate Journey, The, 106–7
  See also perinatal level

Guss, Jeffrey, 228–29

Halifax, Joan, 106–7

Hallelujah Revolution, 67

Hallucinogens, 70

Hallucinogens and Shamanism, 149

"Hallucinogens as Medicine," 10

Harbor-UCLA Medical Center Study, 108–16

Harman, Willis, 136–37

Harner, Michael, 149

Hayes, Charles, 225

Healy, Melissa, 88–89

Heard, Gerald, 29

Heffter Research Institute, 11, 132

Heinrich, Clark, 150

Hendricks, Gay, 212

Hero with a Thousand Faces, The, 173

higher education, 11–12, 216–18

Higher Wisdom, 142, 159

Hillman, D. C. A., 151

Hirshberg, Caryle, 97–99

Hoffman, Edward, 12, 33–34

Hofmann, Albert, 148

Holotropic Mind, The, 47–48

Hood, Ralph, 25, 34, 35, 94, 140, 142

Hruby, Paula Jo, 72

Human Encounter with Death, The, 106

human genome, mapping, 184

"Human Hallucinogen Research: Guidelines for Safety," 76

humanistic education, 212–13

humanities, experimental, 129

human mind
  cognitive-based shifts, 112–13
  enhanced view of, 192
  hidden parameters of, 143–44
  map of, 31, 126, 127, 159–61

Hunsberger, Bruce, 34

Huxley, Aldous, 60, 105

ideas. *See* intellectual endeavors

IgA (salivary immunoglobulin A), 91–92, 95–98

imagery, 92, 96

immune system
  mindbody psychotechnologies for,
    92–94
  overview, 100–101
  peak-experience variable, 90–91
  psychospiritual and psychosocial
    boosts for, 95–97
  salivary immunoglobulin A (IgA)
    measurements, 91–92, 95–98
  spontaneous remission, 89, 97–100
  strengthening, 6, 88–89, 93–94
Inception, 177
ineffability, 27–28
Integral Psychology, 84
intellectual endeavors
  amuses-têtes, 152–58
  multistate ideas, 146–52
  summary, 158
intelligence, improving, 141, 183
Intoxication, 156–57
Island (Huxley), 60
It's a Wonderful Life, 15–16

Jacobson, Bertil, 163
James, William, 18, 19, 69, 122
Johns Hopkins Medical Institute,
    psilocybin study, 8–9, 16–17,
    49–50, 58, 74–76, 78, 226
Johnson, Matthew, 51, 76
Journal of Religion and Health, 94

Kapleau, Philip, 86
Kast, Eric, 106
Katz, Stephen, 84
Kingsley, David, 187
Kleiman, Mark, 58
Kubie, Lawrence, 218–19
Kung, Hans, 62–63

Kurzweil, Ray, 178

Labate, Beatriz, 77
Lancet, The, 8, 9
learning process, 32–33, 210
Lee, Martin, 152
Lerner, Michael, 53–54, 142
leukemia, 88–89
life after death, 30
Limitless, 177
Long Trip, The, 149–50
Lost Civilizations of the Stone Age, The,
    150
"LSD and the Anguish of Dying," 105–6
"LSD and the Enlightenment of Zen," 13
LSD (d-lysergic acid diethylamide)
  Bill Wilson's experience with, 29–30
  Frances Vaughan's experience, 57
  Huxley taking, 105
  impact of, 13
  LSD psychotherapy, 31, 57
  making from microbes, 182
  in psycholytic psychotherapy, 89–90
  relieving pain with, 106
  use in problem solving, 135–36
  why not to put LSD in friend's
    coffee, 226–27
LSD: Doorway to the Numinous, 31,
    66–67, 226
Lyvers, Michael, 53–54, 142

MacLean, Katherine, 51
*Magic Mushrooms in Religion and
    Alchemy*, 150
map of the human mind, 31, 126, 127,
    159–61
MAPS (Multidisciplinary Association for
    Psychedelic Studies), 9, 132, 139–40

marijuana, sacramental use, 89

Maslow, Abraham, 33–34, 52, 63, 212

Master Gene, The, 40–41

materialism, 25–26

Matossian, Mary, 154

Matrix, The, 176–77

Matsunaga, Masahiro, 95

McCann, Una, 75

McKenna, Dennis, 230

MDMA (Ecstasy), 71, 107–8, 140,
181, 226–27

mescaline, 60, 68, 120, 135, 165, 167–68

Metzner, Ralph, 70

Miller, William R., 15–17, 31, 35, 36,
45, 46, 52, 53

mindbody states
anthropologists interest in, 148–49
beyond the singlestate fallacy, 123–24
described, 2, 125
education and, 207–8
mystical experiences as, 2
overview, 124–25
producing new states, 122
psychotechnologies, 92–94
skills transferred to another state, 136
sleeping and dreaming, 210–11
studies, 218
techniques for enhancing, 145
vast and unknown, 179
See also multistate theory

Mithoefer, Michael, 140

Mojeiko, Valerie, 9

money addiction, 39–40

mood (deeply felt, positive), 22–23, 93–94

moral development, 38

Morris, Kelly, 9

*Mosby's Complementary & Alternative
Medicine*, 92

movies, perinatal analysis, 169–77

Mullis, Kary, 135–36, 141

"Multidisciplinary Approaches to
Psychedelic Scholarship," 225

Multidisciplinary Association for
Psychedelic Studies (MAPS), 9,
132, 139–40

multisite studies, 191–92

multistate ideas, 146–52

multistate theory
beyond the singlestate fallacy, 123–24
central multistate question, 128,
208, 214
designing new cognitive processes,
132–33
overview, 120, 121–22, 133–34
psychotechnologies, 126–27
research studies, 130–32
residence, 127–28
theoretical implications, 129–32
See also mindbody states

mushrooms, psychoactive, 154–55, 156

mystical experiences
Bill Wilson's, 27–28, 32
characteristics of, 17–30, 94
contributions to beliefs and
knowledge, 65–69
democratizing, 57–62
as foundation of religion, 56, 62–64
as gift from God, 83
life-changing aspects, 13–14, 83,
85–87
overview, 5–6
as peak experiences, 33–36
POTT MUSIC mnemonic for, 15–17
during psychedelic psychotherapy,
113–14
research on, 94–95

spontaneous remission and, 89, 97–100

theoretical framework for, 83–85

values raised through, 37–38

See also drug-induced mystical
experiences; natural mystical
states; psychedelic-induced
mystical experiences

"Mystical Experiences Occasioned by
the Hallucinogen Psilocybin," 51

"Mystical-type Experiences
Occasioned by Psilocybin," 16–17,
58, 75

mystic fusion, 52

Mysticism, 14

Mysticism and Religious Traditions, 84

Mysticism Scale (Hood), 25, 35, 94,
140, 142

nanotechnology, 184–85

natural mystical states

characteristics of, 17–30

drug-induced states versus, 82–83

long-term effects of, 83, 85–87

psychedelic-induced versus, 16, 17

value shifts from, 45–47

near the end of life

conclusions, 116

Harbor-UCLA Medical Center
Study, 108–15

psychedelic psychotherapy for, 104–8

psychological distress during, 102–3

See also death

Needs Hierarchy (Maslow's), 34, 35

negative emotions, 93–94, 95

Nerurkar, Aditi, 93

"Neuropharmacology of Religious
Experience The," 142

neuropsychology, 190

neuroscience, 179–81

Neurosingularity Project

amplifying intelligence, 183

described, 178–79

genetic leads, 182

insight, intervention, and invention,
183–88

neuroscience leads, 179–81

savant syndrome, 188–90

synthetic biology, 182–83

neurotransmitters, designing, 185–88

Nichols, David, 142

Novotney, Amy, 9

objectivity, 18–20

openness, 51

O'Regan, Brendon, 97–99

organizations, entheogenic, 77–78

Osmond, Humphry, 152

Pahnke, Walter, 73, 94, 139–40

paradigms, inventing, 214–16

paradoxicality of perspective, 17–18

Parker, Alice, 184–85

Pasteur, Louis, 87

Paths Beyond Ego, 84

*Pathways to Higher Consciousness
Beyond the Drug Experience*, 41

PCR (polymerase chain reaction),
135–36

peak experience, 33–36, 90–91

peak performance, 208

perinatal level

analysis, 165–76

Basic Perinatal Memories (BPMs),
164–65

effects of, 161–64

mindbody explorer as hero, 176–77

movie interpretations, 169–77

"Perinatal Roots of Wars, Revolutions, and Totalitarianism, The," 165–66

personal characteristics, highly valued, 47

perspective, paradoxicality of, 17–18

pharmacology, 180–81

philosophy, perinatal, 167–68

Pink Floyd: The Wall, 174–76, 177

Plants of the Gods, 148

poetry, 211

politics, perinatal aspects, 165

polymerase chain reaction (PCR), 135–36

positive emotions, 93–96

positive psychology, 11–12

Positive Psychology, 12

post-traumatic stress disorder, 108, 140

POTT MUSIC mnemonic, 15–17. *See also* mystical experiences

pregnancy, psychedelics and, 227

pride, 39, 41

prize awards, for course development, 230–31

Problem of Pure Consciousness, The, 84

problem solving
  psychedelic, 135–38
  while asleep or dreaming, 210

psilocybin
  benefits for cognitive sciences, 138–39
  current research, 107
  Harbor-UCLA Medical Center Study, 108–16
  Johns Hopkins study, 8–9, 16–17, 49–50, 58, 74–76, 78, 226

"Psilocybin Can Occasion Mystical-type Experiences," 75

"Psychedelic Agents in Creative Problem Solving," 136–37

psychedelic courses
  design awards, 230–31
  teaching, 192
  See also Foundations of Psychedelic Studies course

Psychedelic Drugs Reconsidered, 5, 100–101, 148–49, 223

Psychedelic Explorer's Guide, The, 38, 50–51, 72, 76, 137

psychedelic-induced mystical experiences
  addiction treatments, 29
  Bill Wilson's, 29–30
  characteristics of, 17–30
  described, 3, 6, 81
  natural mystical states versus, 16, 17
  during psychedelic psychotherapy, 113–14
  strengthening the immune system, 6, 88–89, 93–94
  value shifts after, 47–54
  See also drug-induced mystical experiences

Psychedelic Medicine, 7

Psychedelic Psychiatry, 152

psychedelic psychotherapy
  body-based changes, 110–11
  cognitive aspects of, 112–13, 140
  Harbor-UCLA Medical Center Study, 108–16
  mystical experiences during, 113–14
  peak-experience variables, 90–91
  psycholytic, 3, 89–90
  research, 12, 105–8
  treatment sessions, 104–5
  videos and websites, 116–17

Psychedelic Reflections, 181

Psychedelic Renaissance, The, 152

psychedelics
   benefits of, 2, 5–6
   enhancing cognition, 135–41,
      144–45
   as entrances to rich idea minds,
      119–20, 146
   for experimental religious studies,
      139–40
   health-enhancing applications, 7
   history of, 152
   improving intelligence, 141
   introduced to modern Western
      world, 80–81
   long-term effects of, 87
   in medical education, 228
   as psychomagnifiers, 2
   raising values, 37–38
   rediscovery of, 8–11
   reducing the fear of death, 6
   research on, 10–11
   See also entheogens; LSD (d-lysergic
      acid diethylamide)
psychoactive plants, 58, 148, 149–51
Psychology of Religion, 34, 45
psycholytic psychotherapy, 3, 89–90
psychotechnologies
   classroom applications, 208–11
   described, 126–27, 209
   films, 176–77
   mindbody, 92–94
   moving toward super brains, 179
psychotherapists, selecting, 116
psychotherapy. See psychedelic
   psychotherapy

Quantum Change, 15–17, 31, 35, 36,
   45, 46, 52, 53
"Question of Balance," 59

Realms of the Human Unconscious, 173
religion
   mystical experiences as foundation
      of, 56, 62–64
   psychedelic entheogens
      contributions to, 64–78
   text-based placing rite-based, 55,
      56–57, 61, 65, 79
   transition from word-based to
      experience-based, 55, 57–62, 79
Religion, Altered States of Consciousness,
   and Social Change, 148
Religion and Psychoactive Sacraments,
   72
Religions, Values, and Peak Experiences,
   63
religious experiences. See mystical
   experiences
religious studies, experimental, 139–40
research
   multistate theory, 130–32
   mystical experiences, 94–95
   psychedelic psychotherapy, 105–8
   psychedelics, 10–11
"Research on Psychedelics Moves into
   the Mainstream," 9
residence, 127–28
Richards, William, 75, 90, 94
Riedlinger, June, 32
Riedlinger, Thomas, 32, 161–62, 167–68
Ritalin (methylphenidate), 49–50
ritual, entheogenic
   accumulated knowledge, 70–73
   ethics contributions, 76
   experiment-based leads, 73–76
   indigenous rituals, 70
   organizations, 77–78
Roberts, Andy, 152

Roberts, Thomas
  hopes of, 232–34
  "Multidisciplinary Approaches to
    Psychedelic Scholarship," 225
  Psychedelic Medicine, 7
  *Religion and Psychoactive
    Sacraments*, 72
  Second Centering Book, The, 212
  See also Foundations of Psychedelic
    Studies course
Robinson, Monique, 162–63
Ruck, Carl, 150
Rudgley, Richard, 150

Sacred Mushroom Seeker, The, 167
sacredness, 24–27, 49, 89
salivary immunoglobulin A (IgA),
  91–92, 95–98
Samorini, Giorgio, 156–57
Sandison, Roland, 152
Santa's flying reindeer, 155–56
Sarte, Jean Paul, 167
"Sartre's Rite of Passage," 167–68
savant syndrome, 188–90
Schachter-Shalomi, Zalman, 66
Schultes, Richard, 148
Scientific American, 8, 10, 153, 222, 223
Seaman, Gary, 147
Second Centering Book, The, 212
Secret Chief Revealed, The, 70–71, 181
self-actualization, 52–53
Sessa, Ben, 152
set and setting, importance of, 116
seven deadly sins, 39
Sewick, Bruce, 228
shamanism, 147
Shanon, Benny, 67, 130, 143–44, 148,
  214–16, 225

Shlain, Bruce, 152
Siegel, Ronald, 156–57
Singing to the Plants, 228
singlestate fallacy, 123–24
Singularity Is Near, The, 178
skull, human, 187
sleeping and dreaming, 210–11
Smith, Huston, 60, 68, 76, 82, 83, 84, 85
Snow White and the Seven Dwarfs,
  169–70, 173–74, 176
Snyder, Allan, 189
social support, 96–97
Spilka, Bernard, 34
spiritualcompetency (website), 11
spontaneous remission, 89, 97–100
Spontaneous Remission, 97–99
Sternberg, Robert, 141
Stevens, Jay, 152
Stietencron, Heinrich von, 62–63
Stolaroff, Myron, 70–72, 181
Storming Heaven, 152
stress, perinatal, 162–63
stress-reduction techniques, 96
St. Thomas Aquinas, 58–59
suicide, birth experiences and, 163

"Taking Birth Trauma Seriously," 32,
  161–62
Tart, Charles, 84, 85, 123
terminal illness, 101, 102–4
text-based religions, 55, 56–57, 61, 65,
  79
Thanatos to Eros, 181
"Theory of Metamotivation, A," 52
"Theory Z," 34–35
Three Pillars of Zen, The, 86
timelessness, 21, 215
Toward a Psychology of Being, 52

transcendence
  described, 15, 20–21, 24
  difficulties of, 44
  ego death/ego loss, 30, 51
  importance of, 76
  multistate theory of, 133
  near the end of life, 104
  during psychedelic psychotherapy, 114
  self-centeredness reduced, 49
  spontaneous remission and, 100
  values of transcenders, 52–53
transience, 21–22
transpersonal psychology, 20, 35, 94
transpersonal states, 104, 114
Treffert, Darold, 188
Triarchic Mind, The, 141
Tripping, 225
truthfulness, perception of, 19–20
Turning East, 59–60

Ultimate Journey, The, 106–7
unity, 89, 215
urine, psychoactive, 154–55

values
  contributions to ethics, 76
  life values, empathy, and coping with
    stress, 53–54
  lower versus higher, 39–41
  non-egoic, 48–51
  of self-transcenders, 52–53
  shifts after mystical experiences, 45–54
values, problematic
  greed and money addiction, 39–40
  ostentation and, 41–44
  raising, 37–38, 44
  roots of, 39–41

"Values and Beliefs of Psychedelic
    Drug Users," 53–54
Van Dusen, Wilson, 13
Varieties of Anomalous Experience, 123
Varieties of Religious Experience, 18
Vaughan, Frances, 57, 59, 65–66, 84,
    85
videos and websites, 11, 116–17

Wainwright, William, 14
Wallace, Bob, 137–38
Walsh, Roger
  "Entheogens: True or False?" 80
  Higher Wisdom, 142, 159
  Paths Beyond Ego, 84
  Psychedelic Reflections, 181
  using insights gained from mystical
    experiences, 6, 79
  World of Shamanism, The, 80
war, perinatal roots of, 165–67
Wilber, Ken, 84
Wills, Russel, 212
Wilson, Bill, 27–30, 32
Wilson, Edward O., 142–43
Winkelman, Michael, 7, 123, 129
witchcraft persecution, 153–54
womb experiences, 31, 164
World of Shamanism, The, 80
World's Religions, The, 68
Wulff, David, 45, 49

Your Money and Your Brain, 40

Zeff, Leo, 71, 181
Zig Zag Zen, 142
zoology, 155–57
Zweig, Jason, 40

BOOKS OF RELATED INTEREST

Spiritual Growth with Entheogens
Psychoactive Sacramentals and Human Transformation
Edited by Thomas B. Roberts, Ph.D.

The Psychedelic Explorer's Guide
Safe, Therapeutic, and Sacred Journeys
by James Fadiman, Ph.D.

The New Science of Psychedelics
At the Nexus of Culture, Consciousness, and Spirituality
by David Jay Brown

DMT: The Spirit Molecule
A Doctor's Revolutionary Research into the Biology of
Near-Death and Mystical Experiences
by Rick Strassman, M.D.

Inner Paths to Outer Space
Journeys to Alien Worlds through Psychedelics and
Other Spiritual Technologies
*by Rick Strassman, M.D., Slawek Wojtowicz, M.D.,
Luis Eduardo Luna, Ph.D., and Ede Frecska, M.D.*

The Pot Book
A Complete Guide to Cannabis
Edited by Julie Holland, M.D.

Entheogens and the Future of Religion
Edited by Robert Forte

LSD and the Divine Scientist
The Final Thoughts and Reflections of Albert Hofmann
by Albert Hofmann

INNER TRADITIONS • BEAR & COMPANY
P.O. Box 388 • Rochester, VT 05767
1-800-246-8648
www.InnerTraditions.com

Or contact your local bookseller